D0975983

Alzheimer's Activities

Alzheimer's Activities

Hundreds of Activities for Men and Women with Alzheimer's Disease and Related Disorders

Volume 1

B. J. FitzRay

Rayve Productions

Rayve Productions Inc.
Box 726 Windsor CA 95492

Printed in the United States of America

Library of Congress Cataloging-in-Publication Data

FitzRay, B.J.,
   Alzheimer's Activities, Volume 1: Hundreds of Activities for Men and Women with Alzheimer's Disease and Related Disorders / B.J. FitzRay
   p. cm.
   ISBN 1-877810-80-0 (alk. paper)
   1. Alzheimer's disease--Patients--Recreation. 2. Alzheimer's disease--Patients--Rehabilitation. 3. Caregivers. I. Title.

RC523.2 .F585 2001
362.1'96831--dc21

2001019888

To D.C. and V.E.
with deepest love

and

all caregivers of Alzheimer's patients

Note

This book is not intended to provide medical or other professional advice. For specific guidance regarding activities and exercises, contact your family physician or other appropriate healthcare provider. No responsibility can be assumed by the publishers for any loss or damage alleged to be caused directly or indirectly by the information contained in this book.

Approximately 4 million Americans
have Alzheimer's disease.

Seven out of 10 Alzheimer's patients live at home.

Almost 75 percent of their home care
is provided by family and friends.

Three out of four caregivers are women.

A person with Alzheimer's disease
lives an average of 8 years
and as many as 20 or more years
from the onset of symptoms.

—statistics courtesy of the Alzheimer's Association

Why This Book Was Written

When my father, a relatively high functioning 92 year old with Alzheimer's-type dementia, came to live with my husband and me two years ago, we began searching for activities Dad would enjoy, which would increase his feelings of usefulness and self-worth and be appropriate for his skill level. Among the numerous excellent books on Alzheimer's disease, we found many generalized ideas for activities (e.g. "Play an easy game you both will enjoy; work in the garden; help in the kitchen."), but few books provided enough specific recommendations to meet our needs. We also had difficulty finding, evaluating, and shopping for activity resources. In time, mainly through trial and error, we discovered a variety of activities that Dad enjoyed. His life was also enriched by interacting with extended family members and friends who shared these experiences, and their lives were enriched by interacting with him.

Based on our family's personal experiences, and with input from professional and lay caregivers, I compiled the following ideas, suggestions, and activities. I sincerely hope they save you time, give you inspiration, encouragement and insight, and result in more meaningful and positive interactions between you and your mentally impaired loved one, friend or patient.

B.J. FitzRay

Who Should Read This Book?

- Family members caring for Alzheimer's dementia (AD) patients or other mentally impaired patients at home
- Professional healthcare providers and staff working in hospitals, facilities for the mentally impaired, medical offices, clinics
- Alzheimer's day care program providers
- Activity directors for the mentally impaired
- Students who will be working in the healthcare field
- Family members and friends who interact with Alzheimer's patients
- Everyone who wants to learn more about caring for Alzheimer's patients

Why Activities?

Alzheimer's patients benefit greatly from participation in activities, especially those they enjoy. Not surprisingly, caregivers who plan, organize, encourage and share these activities enjoy many of the same benefits. You, the caregiver, may have to stretch your imagination to find appropriate pleasurable activities, or you may discover simple, fun-filled things to do right under your nose. Following are some of the benefits your AD family member may experience from successful activities.

- Enjoy happier daily life
- Increase feelings of self-worth
- Enhance and maintain general health

•Maintain memory
•Enhance and maintain communication skills
•Improve and increase personal relationships
•Preserve family history
•Strengthen and maintain muscles
•Reduce muscle and joint pain
•Increase and maintain flexibility
•Reduce nervous tension
•Decrease pacing and restlessness
•Decrease repetitive behaviors
•Decrease wandering
•Increase nighttime sleep

Who Is Able to Participate in Activities?

Most Alzheimer's patients, until the final stages of the disease, are able to participate in some pleasurable activities. Because each Alzheimer's patient is unique, he or she will respond to activities according to their levels of mental and physical abilities and personal interests. Some Alzheimer's patients have memory impairment but are physically adept. Others suffer from memory impairment and physical disabilities — reduced vision and hearing, back pain, stiff joints, tremors, erratic equilibrium, lack of coordination, muscle weakness, or other difficulties. This book contains suggestions for simple, moderate and moderately complex activities, some of which should be appropriate for your AD family member.

Examples and anecdotes of family experiences are real but names have been changed.

How to Use This Book

This book has been formatted to address both Alzheimer's patients and their caregivers with the primary focus directed to those caring for mentally impaired family members at home. However, much of the information and many of the activities will also prove helpful to professionals working in medical facilities, day care programs, and assisted-living residences.

> NOTE: In this book, the abbreviation "AD" is used as a synonym for Alzheimer's disease, Alzheimer's dementia, and Alzheimer's-demented.

1) Generally, the first sentence of bulleted items suggests an activity for your Alzheimer's (AD) family member or patient.
2) Information and tips following the first sentence are for caregivers.
3) In many sections, there are suggested questions to aid caregivers in conversing meaningfully with AD patients.
4) Historical data is included in some sections to help caregivers more fully understand and appreciate AD patients' backgrounds and possible life experiences and to encourage and facilitate meaningful discussions.
5) Background information on religious holy days and traditional American holidays is intended for those who are unfamiliar with their patients' spiritual or social orientations and life experiences.
6) Resources for products and information are located in the appendix.

Taking Care of the Caregiver

Taking care of a patient with Alzheimer's disease (AD) is a labor or love, and those who assume round-the-clock responsibilities for family members with AD often neglect themselves. <u>Please do not disregard your own needs</u>. You are as important as the patient, and you'll be a healthier, happier, stronger person and caregiver if you maintain your physical, mental, emotional, and spiritual health.

1) **Don't try to do everything**. No one can do it all, and many people who thought they could collapsed or died trying. Simplify life and do only what is truly necessary.

2) **Learn all you can about Alzheimer's disease**. You will be better prepared for caregiving responsibilities and important decision-making.

3) **Maintain a sense of humor**. In erratic but non-crisis situations, choose to smile. A positive attitude softens life's rough spots.

4) **Participate in an AD support group**. You are not alone in what you face. Other AD caregivers understand your challenges and will provide resource information, caregiving tips and encouragement.

5) **Ask for and accept help from others**. When you allow others to help you, you bless them with "acceptional" love.

6) **Reward yourself periodically**. Have a massage, eat a hot-fudge sundae, read a good book, or relax in a bubble bath. You deserve it!

7) **Make time for yourself regularly**. Get away from

the house and caregiver responsibilities — have lunch with a friend, go to a movie, relax at the beach, play a round of golf.

8) **Get adequate sleep**. If nighttime sleep is interrupted, take naps during the day whenever possible. Consult your doctor regarding excessive loss of sleep.

9) **Learn about and use community services**. Many local programs designed to help stressed families will make your life easier.

10) **Exercise regularly**. Go for walks, take an aerobics class, go bowling, work out with a videotape.

11) **Have regular medical checkups**. Take care of routine health concerns, and talk openly to your doctor about physical and emotional stresses and any depression you may be experiencing. If your doctor is not sensitive to your needs as an AD caregiver, find a doctor who is.

Tips for Successful Activities

The following techniques have proved helpful to many caregivers in facilitating activities with Alzheimer's patients.

1) Accept your loved one as he or she is.
2) Plan ahead and organize activities before involving your mentally impaired family member.
3) Remember K I S S — **Keep It Simple, Sweetheart**.
4) Be calm and encouraging.
5) Speak gently and reassuringly.
6) Focus on your loved one. Make eye contact. Use

his or her name and terms of endearment. This helps get their attention and maintain their focus.

7) Don't try to teach new skills. Concentrate on old, familiar abilities.

8) Laugh and smile frequently. Your body language is important. Pat a shoulder. Give a hug.

9) Don't argue. It's better to change the subject or redirect his or her attention.

10) Maintain a positive attitude. Do not talk to or treat your mentally impaired loved one like an inferior person. He or she is a living being, God's creation, deserving of love and respect.

11) If agitation and tension build during an activity, take a break or abandon the activity altogether.

12) Display art and craft projects where they can be viewed and praised.

13) Once you've found activities that make your loved one happy, consider settling into a routine, repeating the activities systematically. Don't worry about his or her becoming bored; the routine is likely to foster an added sense of security.

An Invitation

We invite readers to send us descriptions of successful activities you have tried, problems confronted, and anecdotes about your experiences. All submissions received become the property of Rayve Productions and may be considered for possible inclusion in future editions of this book. Forward submissions or contact the publisher at the following locations.

Rayve Productions
P.O. Box 726
Windsor, CA 95492
rayvepro@aol.com; 1-707-838-6200

Acknowledgments

♥ Honor and glory to God Almighty, who is the heart and soul of my life. He guides me daily and has taught me to recognize His blessings in all circumstances.

♥ Heartfelt gratitude to the Alzheimer's patients I have been privileged to know — family members, friends and casual acquaintances — whose life experiences were the inspiration for this book.

♥ My deepest appreciation to the professional and family caregivers who served as my mentors and shared personal stories, insights and sound advice.

♥ Sincerest thanks to the national Alzheimer's Association for information and statistics; and Barry Reisberg, M.D., geriatric psychiatrist and professor, New York University School of Medicine, for allowing me to reproduce his chart on the functional stages of Alzheimer's disease.

♥ Bouquets to the staff at Primrose Special Alzheimer's Living facility (Santa Rosa, California), especially Executive Director William Keck; Day Club Director Hortencia Haro, A.C.; Wellness Director Vannessa Breedlove, L.V.N.II; and former Day Club Director Heather Sevigny, A.C.; for their examples of exceptional patient care and for research assistance.

♥ Many thanks to those who contributed their time and expertise in reviewing and fine-tuning my manuscript:

Karen Fraire, M.A., medical social services; Cynthia M. Thomas, M.S., CCC-SLP, speech/language pathologist; Susan Pringle-Cohan, M.A., exercise physiologist and writer; Anne Muller, A.C., transitional care center activities director; Ellen DeLa Vega, R.N., assisted-living facility; Rabbi Jonathan Slater, Congregation Beth Ami (Santa Rosa, California), whose recommendations greatly enhanced the sections on Jewish holy days; Sharon Traeger, who helped me better understand Jewish history and religion; and Gayle Mallison, who enthusiastically helped me identify and adapt activities for my father.

♥Finally, I am profoundly grateful to my husband, Norm, and my family for their unfailing love and support during my work on this project and always.

Contents

Activities

Activities

Activity Books

Books designed for young children are often ideal for use by mentally impaired men and women, provided they do not recognize and feel embarrassed by the for-children format. Test the waters by adding activity books to other material they are reading or looking through, and ask them how they like the new books. You might also sit beside your family member and work on a couple of activities in a children's book, stating enthusiastically how much fun you're having, then invite him or her to try an activity with you.

❏Fill in coloring book illustrations using crayons or felt-tipped pens.
❏Discover the ease of paint-with-water books.
❏Enjoy follow-the-dot books.
❏Have fun with paint-by-number books

"I was sure my mother, a former elementary school teacher, would realize she was coloring in a children's book, but she didn't."

"Uncle Rubin wouldn't try any creative project. 'I'd just mess it up,' he'd say glumly. Then one day he became interested in a dot-to-dot book his six-year-old niece was enjoying, and she let him finish a picture she had started. After that, Uncle Rubin was an avid dot-to-dotter. He didn't always follow the numbers correctly, but

*he didn't notice the errors, and we didn't
tell him, so he felt he was successful. "*

Advent (December 1-24)

*Advent is derived from the Latin word "adventus" (a
coming) and honors the coming of Christ. On the old,
traditional Christian calendar, Advent varies from year
to year, beginning on the fourth Sunday before Christmas
and ending on Christmas Eve. In earlier centuries, it
was a solemn time observed by fasting and praying.
Today, Americans celebrate the season from December
1 to December 24 using Advent calendars and other
fun-filled ways to count down the days until Christmas.
In many families, children receive a small gift each day.*

☐Attend an Advent service at church.

☐Create a Christmas scene to mark the days of
Advent. **Caregiver**: Each day, have your AD
family member glue on one of 24 cutouts or
stickers — Mary, Joseph, angels, wise men,
shepherds, animals, stars, etc. On Christmas
Day, place Baby Jesus in the manger.

☐Decorate a small Christmas tree with a mini-
ornament. **Caregiver**: Provide a variety or 25
doves, balls, angels, bows, etc., one for each
day of Advent.

☐Read a portion of scripture or an inspirational
devotion each day of Advent.

☐Read an Advent story.

☐Hand-craft small gifts to give to children during Advent.

☐Say a prayer for a different, special person in your life each day of Advent.

☐Share an Advent memory from days gone by.

☐Use a colorful Advent calendar to mark each day before Christmas.

Airplanes/Aviation

Many older Americans remember the excitement of America's first airplanes. Brothers Wilbur and Orville Wright, recognized as the fathers of 20th century aviation, built and successfully flew the first "flying machine." Orville Wright (who lived until 1948) piloted the craft 120 feet at Kitty Hawk, North Carolina in December 1903. In 1927, Charles Lindbergh flew the first solo nonstop transatlantic flight from New York to Paris in 33½ hours. In 1927, Amelia Earhart was the first woman to cross the Atlantic. Both Lindbergh and Earhart became instant celebrities.

☐Attend a presentation by an aviation historian.

☐Collect and display miniature aircraft.

☐Hang an airplane mobile from the ceiling.

☐Look through a picture book on airplanes and aviation history.

☐Put together an airplane jigsaw puzzle.

☐Read a story or book about the Wright brothers, Charles Lindbergh, Amelia Earhart, Wiley

Post, or others.

❐Record stories about your air industry work or flight experiences on audio- or videotape.

❐Talk about airplane history. When did you see your first airplane? What did you think and feel? What stories did your parents tell you about the first airplanes? Were you frightened by the first jets and the loud sonic booms? What do you remember most about the Wright brothers, Wilbur and Orville? Charles Lindberg? Amelia Earhart?

❐Talk about your flying experiences. Have you flown in an airplane? How old were you on your first flight and where did you go? Have you piloted an airplane? When and where? Were you a military or a civilian pilot? Did you own your own plane? What was your most exciting flight? Your favorite trip?

❐Talk about your air industry career or work experiences. What type work did you do in the air industry? Was it a military or a civilian job? How and where were you trained to do this work? Why was this work impor-tant? Where did you work? How many years did you work there? What did you like best about your work? What did you like least?

❐Visit an air museum.

❐Visit an airport to watch airplanes in action.

❐Watch a movie about flight. (*See reference section for suggestions.*)

Antiques & Memorabilia

If you don't recognize an object in an antique or secondhand store, ask your elderly AD family member to help you. Often, he or she will know what the item is and share an anecdote about its use in days gone by.

☐ Choose an antique or collectible item in your home (music box, stereopticon, china figurine, canning jar, cigar humidor, handmade lace collar, harmonica, pocket knife, etc.). What are your earliest or favorite memories about the collectible?

☐ Eat a meal or snack using heirloom or favorite old china, linens, or teapot.

☐ Visit antique stores, and talk about old, familiar items. What is it? How was it used? Did your family have one?

> *"I had no idea what the loosely woven, flat metal object was, but Aunt Ida did. 'That's a pot scrubber. Back when I was a child, my mother used one. Scouring pads hadn't been invented.'"*

> *"Although she has Alzheimer's disease, Cousin Bernice has not lost her sense of humor. On a recent trip to an antique store, she announced with a chuckle that she is older than most of the antiques we were looking at."*

Aquariums/Fish Tanks

Few things are as relaxing as an aquarium filled with beautifully colored fish swimming gracefully among water plants. Knowing this, doctors and other health-care professionals have placed aquariums in their offices and facilities for many years to help ease patient stress. Aquariums in the home are also calming, and a well-filtered tank with hearty fish is relatively easy to maintain. Seek advice from an aquarium professional before setting up your system and buying fish.

☐ Add water to the aquarium.

☐ Clean the aquarium. (Caregivers have told me that men especially enjoy helping with this task.)

☐ Feed the fish. **Caregiver**: Monitor this activity so your fish are not overfed and die.

☐ Go to the library and browse through books on aquariums and fish.

☐ Enjoy a faux fish tank with plastic fish. **Caregiver**: These tanks provide the relaxing aquarium atmosphere without the responsibilities of live fish. You'll find faux fish tanks at varying prices in department, variety and import stores, and through novelty catalogs.

☐ Turn on the aquarium light at specific times.

☐ Visit a pet shop to buy fish. **Caregiver**: Allow enough time to leisurely view the fish and decide which ones to take home.

☐ Watch a video featuring fish in natural settings,

especially colorful fish similar to those in your aquarium.

Arbor Day (Date varies)

Arbor Day was the idea of Mr. J. Sterling Morton of Nebraska, where the holiday was first observed on April 10, 1872. In the first year, more than 1,000,000 trees were planted in Nebraska. Arbor Day is now observed in every state and in some foreign countries on a variety of dates from December through May, depending upon regional climate and the best time for planting.

❑Create a card game with magazine pictures of trees or tree scenes. **Caregiver**: Cut the pictures in half and glue them to cards. For permanent use, laminate the cards. Spread the cards out on a table and have your AD family member match as many as possible.

If you make enough cards (56 is standard but two can play with fewer), two or more people can play a matching game. Deal seven cards to each player, placing the remaining cards (the "log pile") face down in the middle of the table. Players match as many trees as they can from cards they are holding, placing trees (their "forest") face up on the table. Then, they take turns drawing additional cards from the log pile, adding trees to their forest as they match cards. When all the cards have been drawn, the player with the most trees in his or her forest wins.

☐Cut out magazine pictures of trees, and glue or paste a "forest" on a sheet of paper.

☐Cut out magazine pictures of things made of wood. **Caregiver**: Help your family member glue or paste the pictures on cards and guess what kind of tree each object is made from.

☐Find several wood objects around the house made of various types of wood — a cedar box, wooden spoon, pine cabinet, mahogany curio shelf, oak table. Look at the beautiful grain and finish on the wood. Feel the texture. Smell the fragrance. Do any of these objects bring back pleasant memories?

☐Gather and press several tree leaves.

☐Go to the library and look through a book about trees.

☐Have your picture taken beside your favorite tree.

☐Laminate fresh tree leaves to maintain their beauty. **Caregiver**: Your AD family member can keep the leaves as a collection or use them for decorations.

☐Look through family photographs for scenes with trees. What types of trees are they? Where was the picture taken? What memories does it bring back?

☐Paint a picture of a tree.

☐Plant a seedling tree.

☐Read poetry or short stories about trees, or write your own.

☐Rest in a hammock under a big tree.

☐Sit awhile under a shady tree, eating cookies and drinking lemonade.

☐Take a stroll along a tree-lined street, especially when trees are blooming.

☐Talk about happy childhood memories of climbing trees, favorite trees, and swings. Did you climb trees as a child? What was the tallest tree you climbed? Did you swing in your yard, at a neighbor's home, at school, or at a park? What type swings did you enjoy as a child — metal swing set, single rope swing, tire swing or other?

☐Tour a nursery that specializes in trees, or a tree farm.

☐Travel around town (via car, bus, taxi, etc.) and look for the tallest, biggest in circumference or oldest tree.

☐Visit a lumber yard and collect several types of wood samples. Look at the beautiful grain, feel the texture, and smell the fragrance.

> *"Harmon smiled and grew misty eyed when he smelled a piece of freshly cut pine. The fragrance reminded him, he said, of his childhood when he and his father hiked to nearby hills to gather firewood for the winter."*

Armed Forces Day
(Third Saturday in May)

This holiday replaced several other military-related holidays: Army Day in April, Air Force Day in September, and Navy Day in October.

☐Attend a local parade.

☐Display the American flag.

☐Listen to John Philip Souza or other march music.

☐Read a fun-filled book or story about military adventures.

☐Talk about your military service. In which branch of the military did you serve? What was your rank? How old were you? Where in the world did you travel? Did you fight in a war? What were your duties?

☐Watch a humorous video or television program with a military theme — Sgt. Bilko; Gomer Pyle, USMC; Francis the Talking Mule, or others. **Caregiver**: Although there are numerous military-themed videos available for purchase or rent from stores, or by borrowing from libraries, select them with caution, if at all. Many contain violent scenes which may frighten or agitate your AD family member or patient, and violence depicted in recently released war films is especially graphic.

☐Wear an American flag pin on your collar.

Art

Art is the personal expression of beauty, and artistic projects are as varied and unique as the individuals who create them. The following easy-to-do projects are merely a sampling of the endless possibilities in art. Patients and caregivers with art experience may prefer to work on more advanced projects.

☐Attend an art exhibit. **Caregiver**: Professional and amateur exhibits are available throughout the year. Some charge an admission fee but many, like those held in libraries and civic centers, are free. Check your newspaper for dates and other information.

☐Brush a vibrant scene with watercolors. **Caregiver**: Use watercolor paper for best results.

☐Buy and color a paint-by-number picture. **Caregiver**: Kits, from simple to complex, are widely available. Start with a simple design.

☐Color or paint geometric patterns. **Caregiver**: Design the patterns yourself or buy a book of patterns to fill in.

☐Create a multicolored "stained glass" mosaic by tearing small pieces of tissue paper and pasting them on construction paper.

☐Create a picture with finger paints.

☐Fill in colors on a fuzzy art poster. **Caregiver**: The background is black and very forgiving of artistic slips of the brush or pen. Kits from Western Graphics Corporation are available in a variety of sizes. I recommend medium felt-tipped pens.

"Of all the things he has tried, Grandpa likes his fuzzy posters of flowers best. After he colors them, he gives them as gifts to his lady friends."

☐Draw a picture with pastel chalk.
☐Mold a figure or object with modeling clay.
☐Observe artists working in an art class.
☐Take an art class.
☐Tour an art museum.
☐Try freehand artwork using black-lead pencils, colored pencils, pens and paints.
☐Use crayons to fill in coloring book pictures.
  Caregiver: Choose subjects that will appeal to your family member or patient from among the many children's coloring books widely available.
☐Visit an art gallery.
☐Visit an arts and crafts store to look for new projects and supplies.

TIP: For an absorbent, quick-as-a-wink shirt coverup, secure a bath towel around your crafter's neck with an elastic ironing board strap. The towel will stay securely in place with the strap's strong metal clips.

Audiotapes/CDs

A portable audiotape- or CD player will provide many hours of listening pleasure for your AD family member. I recommend a machine small enough to carry easily so he or she can listen to music or stories while working, exercising, and relaxing.

☐ Alphabetize by title, musician or lyricist the audiotapes and CDs in your collection, arranging them on a shelf or in a storage case.

☐ Label your personal audiotapes and CDs with your name, writing with a permanent marking pen directly on the case, tape or a self-sticking label, or use a label gun.

☐ Listen to books or music on tape. **Caregiver**: Buy taped books and music in stores or borrow them from libraries. If your family member is hard of hearing, try using a headset so you can increase volume without disturbing others and to block out distracting sounds in the room.

☐ Keep a record (A spiral bound tablet works well.) of your tapes and CDs. It's fun to review your collection and make choices from the list.

☐ Number tapes and CDs in your collection. **Caregiver**: Sometimes it's easier to remember a number than a title.

☐ Record family facts, anecdotes and stories. **Caregiver**: Many audiotape recorders are voice activated, so you can set them up unobtrusively near your loved one, and when she speaks, her words will be recorded. When no one is speaking, the device shuts off.

❏Remove audiotapes from plastic holders and insert them in the player. When they have finished playing, return them to their plastic holders and to their storage unit.

❏Select audiotapes and CDs to listen to.

❏Visit a store with a sizeable inventory of audiotapes and CDs and buy one or two favorites. **Caregiver**: Allow adequate time for leisurely browsing.

Automobiles

The first Americans to make and operate a successful gasoline automobile were brothers Charles and Frank Duryea in 1893, in Springfield, Massachusetts. In 1896 the Duryea Motor Wagon Company produced 13 automobiles.

In 1899 Ransom Olds founded the Olds Motor Vehicle Company, in Lansing, Michigan, selling 400 vehicles in 1901 and ten times that number in 1903.

Henry Ford is recognized as the father of mass produced, low-cost autos. In 1908 Ford sold more than 10,000 Model T's and some 75,000 in 1912. Most old-timers remember the popular Model T.

❏Attend a local car show.

"On our way shopping, Jimmy spotted classic cars on display in a parking lot. We stopped and he happily roamed from one to another, telling all sorts of stories about cars he and his family had owned."

☐Collect and display miniature automobiles.
☐Go for a ride. **Caregiver**: Whether in the city or country, an automobile ride will be enjoyed. Talk about the passing scene and stop to look at points of interest.

"Bernie's focus had been limited to straight ahead for months, but after several drives where we stopped to look at brilliant fall vineyards, houses under construction, and children at play, Bernie began to turn his head and look out the window more often, even when we weren't stopped."

☐Look at picture books of automobiles, especially those that document automobile history.
☐Read the children's book *Link Across America, The Story of the Lincoln Highway*. **Caregiver**: This story, illustrated with many drawings and photographs, brings back fond memories of life during the 1920s and '30s.
☐Share stories about the cars in your life. **Caregiver**: Virtually every person has interesting stories to tell about automobiles, whether they ever drove or not.

❏Talk about your driving experience. Who taught you how to drive? How old were you? What kind of car did you first drive? Did it have a stick shift or an automatic transmission? What was the first car you owned? Was it given to you or did you work to earn money to buy it? What were the roads like? How fast did you drive? Did you ever have an accident? What is your favorite car?

"Grandma Daisy shyly confessed that in the 1940s, she was once stopped for speeding. However, when the patrolman got out of his car and approached her, she drove off quickly and he didn't catch her."

❏Visit an automobile museum.
❏Visit an automobile showroom.
❏Visit the library and borrow an easy-to-read book about automobiles.

Babies

Many caregivers report that Alzheimer's patients enjoy babies and young children. Perhaps they are reminded of their own childhood, or perhaps they feel more relaxed interacting with the uncomplicated minds and unconditional love of youngsters. If you have no babies or young children in your home, invite friends who have them to visit.

☐Fold baby blankets and diapers.
☐Hold a baby or toddler.
☐Stuff homemade toys.
☐Watch youngsters splash in a tub or wading pool.
☐Wind musical swings and watch baby rock.
☐Wind musical toys and give them to baby.

"More than 30 years ago, my friend, Nancy, asked if I would mind if Grandma Hendrickson held my newborn son. Watching the joy on the face of that nearly blind, wisp of a woman as she rocked and stroked my baby is a memory I'll never forget."

"Gayle brings her young grandchildren, Taylor and Justin, with her when she visits Uncle Fred. They adore the undivided attention of the gentle man who holds them on his lap, shares his crayons, and plays balloon toss with them."

"Viola suffers from aphasia, but three-year-old Patsy carried on an enthusiastic 'conversation' with her for the better part of a morning. Patsy shared her favorite doll and kitten, which Viola caressed affectionately while she chattered unintelligibly, her face happy and expressive. Patsy responded to 'questions' and 'comments' as if she understood exactly what Viola was saying. Later, Patsy commented, 'Mrs. Viola is lots of fun to play with . . . even if she does speak another language.'"

Birthdays

Whether it is your birthday, the birthday of someone you love and care for, or that of another friend or family member, you can celebrate the day with joy and fun-filled activities.

☐ Attend a birthday party.

☐ Bake and decorate a birthday cake.

☐ Blow bubbles with bubble fluid.

☐ Blow out the candles on your birthday cake.

☐ Call a birthday "boy" or "girl" to wish him or her a happy birthday.

☐ Create a collage or album of pictures taken during your life. Label the pictures and share happy memories of bygone years.

☐ Curl ribbon.

☐ Go for a birthday ride in the car.

☐ Go to a dessert shop for a birthday ice cream sundae, soda, pie, cake or other celebration sweet.

☐ Go to a restaurant for a birthday meal. **Caregiver**: Choose a restaurant that provides free dessert (Some also sing "Happy Birthday.") for the birthday celebrant, and call ahead to arrange the surprise.

☐ Help plan and host a birthday party.

☐ Invite a couple of friends over for tea and cookies or cake.

☐ Look through a scrapbook or collection of old birthday cards. Share happy memories.

☐Make gift wrap paper. **Caregiver**: Use large
   sheets of plain paper and help your AD family
   member decorate them with stencils, paint,
   stickers, felt-tipped pens, or stamps. Choose a
   theme appropriate for the birthday — cars,
   pets, sports, books, cosmetics, jewelry, nature,
   cartoons — and cut pictures from magazines
   to glue on the paper.
☐Open cards and gifts.
☐Put bows and ribbon on packages.
☐Put candles on the birthday cake.
☐Sing the traditional "Happy Birthday" song.
☐Talk about happy birthdays. How old are you?
   What is your favorite birthday memory? Did
   you have birthday parties when you were a
   child? What were they like? What was your
   favorite birthday present?
☐Throw confetti and streamers.
☐Wear a party hat.

Books

*Books are treasures that can be enjoyed even after a
mind isn't sharp any longer. Your AD family member or
patient may prefer to be read to some or all of the time.
Select books appropriate to his or her interests, and, if
vision is failing, look for volumes with large type.*

☐Browse through special interest books, magazines and catalogs — auto, collectibles, farm,

fishing, flowers, garden seeds, hunting, pets, stitchery or others.

☐Buy a book to give as a gift.

☐Choose a recipe from a cookbook for a meal. **Caregiver**: Cookbooks with many colorful photographs are most helpful.

☐Dust your books.

☐Enjoy one or more of the books from the *Little House on the Prairie* series. **Caregiver**: Try reading a chapter each day. Discuss with your AD family member how life was long ago, or how it has changed. Was life better then or now? What was best about the "old days?" What is his or her favorite memory of long ago? What stories did parents or grandparents tell about their childhoods?

> *"I had a hard time reading* Little House on the Prairie *to Papa Johnson because he stopped me so often to describe in detail how his childhood compared to the story."*

☐Get inspiration from spiritual devotionals.

☐Listen to a story or book read to you by a child or teenager.

☐Look through old children's storybooks or schoolbooks. **Caregiver**: Especially good are books similar to those your loved one may have read as a child.

☐Nurture your spirit by reading the Bible.

☐Organize your favorite books and magazines on a special shelf.

☐Read a children's book or story to a child.

☐Renew personal pride through the writing and photos in journalist Tom Brokaw's books, *The Greatest Generation ($24.95)* and *The Greatest Generation Speaks ($19.95)*. **Caregiver**: These excellent books focus on the heroism and survival of the men and women who fought in World War II.

☐Relax with poetry. **Caregiver**: Select poetry styles that will appeal to your AD family member. Don't overlook children's poetry. The collected verses of Robert Lewis Stevenson and many other child-oriented works are enjoyable at any age.

☐Reminisce with Norman Rockwell picture books. **Caregiver**: Colorful and happy, Rockwell's illustrations present an idealized picture of American life in days past. People of all ages enjoy the pictures and many AD patients are stimulated to talk about their life experiences. Fortunately, numerous Rockwell books are available at libraries, bookstores, online, and in used-book stores. You may even have one or two in your home library.

☐Share a favorite book or story with a friend.

☐Stamp or write your name on an inside front page of your books.

❒Talk about books and reading. What is your favorite book? What subjects do you enjoy? How old were you when you learned to read? What books, magazines and newspapers did your family read when you were growing up?

❒Use a Book Buddy® pillow to support your book while reading.

❒Visit your local library regularly.

Camping

Not everyone enjoys roughing it, but if your AD family member does, go for it! Even with a walker or wheelchair, camping can be fun. Plan ahead, check out facilities, and make reservations. Select a location with easy access to the campground and toilet accommodations, preferably an area with wide, level paths for leisurely strolls, sunny and shady areas for daydreaming, and a lake, river, or seashore.

❒Browse through the visitors' center.

❒Buy a souvenir in the gift shop.

❒Doze under the trees in a hammock.

> *"My dad's favorite activity is camping and although he's been wheelchair-bound for several years, our family continues to pitch tents or rent rustic cabins every summer. Dad says these adventures are what makes life worth living."*

☐Fish in a lake or river. **Caregiver**: If your family member uses a cane, walker or wheelchair, call ahead to make sure the fishing area is accessible and safe.

☐Go to park rangers' campfire programs.

☐Mail a postcard card to a friend or relative.

☐Make a list or keep a journal of fun things you do while camping. Refer to it later to refresh happy memories.

☐Pose while someone takes your picture or videotapes you enjoying your camping trip.

☐Read a book about the flora and fauna of the area.

☐Play games — cards, board games, or toss a ball around.

☐Roast hot dogs or toast marshmallows and s'mores in the campfire.

☐Set the camp table at mealtime.

☐Sing favorite old songs around the campfire.

☐Stroll through the recreation area on foot or "cruise" in a vehicle.

☐Sweep out the tent or cabin.

☐Talk about your camping experiences. Did you go camping when you were a child? Family camping? Boy Scouts or Girl Scouts? Campfire Girls? YMCA? Church? Where did you camp? What is your favorite camping memory?

☐Tell stories.

☐Wash or dry dishes.

Canes, Walkers & Wheelchairs

Dress up canes, walkers, and wheelchairs to add vitality to daily life and special occasions.

☐Clean or polish your walker or wheelchair.
☐Decorate canes, walkers and wheelchairs.
Caregiver: This easy-to-do, creative activity adds pleasure to everyday happenings and a little glamour to special occasions.

> *"We hung bells from Dad's walker so we could hear where he was, especially when he wandered at night. To our surprise, he loved the 'pretty jingle bells' and wanted to add more."*

> *"Myra Belle didn't want to attend her granddaughter's wedding using a cane, but when it was decorated with pink ribbon and flowers to match her dress, she proudly walked down the aisle and enjoyed many compliments at the reception."*

Card Games

To make card handling easier, buy large-sized cards and/or a card holder. Some of the following card games should be ideal for you and your AD family member to play together. Adjust the rules as necessary to ensure positive self-esteem.

☐Enjoy *Go Fish*.

☐Experience *Finding My Family*. **Caregiver**: In sets of three or four, photocopy or computer scan photographs of familiar relatives (and pets). Attach to playing cards, label boldly with family members' names, and laminate. Follow playing rules for Go Fish or Old Maid.

☐*Match the Pictures*. (see description on page 5, Arbor Day) **Caregiver**: Make your own cards or buy them.

☐Play *Battle* or *War*.

☐Relax with *Old Maid*.

> TIP: Many types of card activities are available through educational, toy and variety stores, online, and through catalogs from companies like Elder Press and Super Duper Publications.

Catalogs

Most of us receive more catalogs than we care to have, but they can be excellent resources for your AD family member. Browsing through catalogs is a pleasurable pastime, and it's fun to receive a product through the mail. Whatever the interest, there's sure to be a catalog (probably several) catering to it. To find specific catalogs, look for ads in magazines or ask your reference librarian for assistance. Following are some favorite catalog types recommended by caregivers.

☐Arts and crafts

☐Baby products
☐Books
☐Clothing
☐Dog and cat supplies
☐Farm and farm-related products
☐Fishing and hunting gear
☐Food
☐Greeting cards
☐Jewelry
☐Novelty items
☐Puzzles and games
☐Sewing supplies
☐Sports equipment
☐Stationery and related supplies
☐Flower and vegetable seeds
☐Tools
☐Toys
☐Yard and garden supplies and equipment

Children

"We need love's tender lessons taught,
As only weakness can;
God hath his small interpreters;
The child must teach the man."

—John Greenleaf Whittier

☐Enjoy greeting cards, letters and pictures from
children. **Caregiver**: If you have a child or
grandchild in school, contact his or her

teacher and request student-created greetings. This can be a very rewarding class activity.

"On his 93rd birthday, Grandpa Claxton was surprised by dozens of greeting cards created by his great-granddaughter Serena's Christian school classmates. Each card quoted a Bible verse and a unique thought (One said, 'How does it feel to be so old?') and delightful illustrations. Grandpa keeps the cards on his night table and reads them frequently."

❑Listen to books or stories read by children. **Caregiver**: Reading aloud is pleasurable to adults and is great reading practice for children. Remember, a youngster doesn't have to be a first-rate reader to bring enjoyment to those who have difficulty reading.

❑Play table games with children. **Caregiver**: Encourage children in your family to play games with mentally impaired adults.

"Aunt Liz wasn't interested in playing games until ten-year-old Anna introduced her to Old Maid and Fish. 'Anna's cards' soon became Aunt Liz's favorite pastime."

❑Work on arts and crafts projects with children.

"Great-aunt Ann's favorite painting partner is two-year-old Rachel. Each delights

in the other's splashes of color and free-form designs. "

Children's Day
(Second Sunday in June)

The first Children's Day was observed by the Methodist Episcopal Church in 1868, and was later adopted by other churches. The celebration is thought to have originated in Europe long before 1868, however, with children traditionally carrying flowering branches to church on May Day.

❑Attend a church service dedicated to children.

❑Bake and deliver cookies to neighborhood children.

❑Enjoy creative play with "Little People" cards and pictures. **Caregiver**: With your AD family member, cut out magazine pictures of babies and young children and paste them on cards or sheets of paper. Take turns naming the babies and children. Describe what you think one or more of the children is doing or thinking, or tell a story about him or her.

❑Go to a happy, G-rated movie with a child.

❑Invite a child to watch favorite old cartoons or films with you. **Caregiver**: Buy or rent videos (Tom & Jerry, Mickey Mouse), or animated feature films (*Bambi, Cinderella, Snow White and the Seven Dwarfs*).

☐Recite a poem or verse learned in childhood.
☐Say a special prayer for a child or children.
☐Sing a favorite children's song.
☐Talk about your childhood. Did your family celebrate Children's Day? What things made you feel special as a child? What things did you do for your children to make them feel special? What was your favorite children's story?
☐Visit a family with children.
☐Watch a Shirley Temple video.

Chinese New Year (Date varies)

Chinese-Americans celebrate this ancient holiday in traditional ways by remembering ancestors, repaying debts, giving gifts, feasting, and warding off evil spirits. The color red, which signifies joy and luck, and dragons are popular during this season. At midnight celebrants drive away any lingering evil spirits from the old year with firecrackers, noise makers, and by waving red ribbons, flags and banners.

☐Attend a parade or watch one on television.
☐Call someone to wish him or her a *Gung Hay Fat Choi!* (Happy New Year!).
☐Count lucky money and put it in red envelopes.
☐Create a New Year banner. **Caregiver**: Have

your AD family member color a preprinted picture (or his or her own design) of a zodiac animal, bamboo, firecrackers, flowers, lanterns, red envelopes, panda, or other symbols. Glue the finished picture to a large sheet of red construction paper, punch holes in upper corners, attach a gold ribbon, and display.

☐Give a "lucky plant" to a family member or friend. **Caregiver**: You'll find jade plants, bamboo, money trees, angel flowers, ginseng and other lucky plants at local nurseries and through the Internet.

☐Give a traditional red envelope containing "lucky money" to a family member or friend.

☐Help prepare food for a New Year feast.

☐Invite a friend over for tea and cookies.

☐Listen to Chinese music.

☐Look at family photographs of past Chinese New Year celebrations. **Caregiver**: Identify and record people, places and dates in the photos, and add significant comments.

☐Make or buy sweet treats and give as gifts.

☐Read a book or story about Chinese New Year, culture, or a famous Chinese man or woman.

☐Share a story about an ancient superstition.

☐Tell a Chinese folktale to a child.

☐Talk about past Chinese New Year experiences. What is your favorite New Year memory? How did your family celebrate when you were a child? What was your favorite gift?

Lunar New Year Dates		
Year	Day	Animal Sign
2001	January 24	Snake
2002	February 12	Horse
2003	February 1	Ram
2004	January 22	Monkey
2005	February 9	Rooster

Christmas (December 25)

December 25 is the day Christians commemorate the birth of Jesus Christ, their Savior, and it is also the day most Americans traditionally decorate Christmas trees, exchange gifts, and feast with family members. For many people, Christmas is the happiest time of the year, and few holidays offer so many opportunities for simple, satisfying interaction with your AD family member or patient.

☐ Add touches of glitter — using glue-glitter or glitter sprinkled on glue — to purchased greeting cards.

☐ Arrange flowers and candles on tables.

☐ Attend church services and programs during December — Christmas Eve, and/or Christmas Day.

☐ Attend community or school musical programs.

☐ Bake and decorate cookies and bread.

☐ Browse through Christmas catalogs.

☐ Curl ribbon.

☐Decorate the Christmas tree.

☐Drape garlands on stairways and fireplace mantels.

☐Dress up in festive red and green clothing and holiday sweaters.

☐Drink hot or cold cider and nibble cookies, candy, candied apples, and popcorn.

☐Drive or walk through "Christmas Tree Lane." **Caregiver**: Locate your area's most festive neighborhood and, if it won't be upsetting to your AD family member, go after dark.

☐Embelish Christmas card envelopes using rubber stamps and ink pads or glue-on stamps.

☐Fill a bowl with fragrant potpourri.

☐Glue miniature decorations — fruit, toys, candy, skates, sleds, snowmen — on a Christmas wreathe.

☐Go to a holiday movie.

☐Go to a performance of the Nutcracker ballet.

☐Handcraft gifts for family members and friends or for holiday bazaars.

☐Hang stockings on the mantle.

☐Hang strings of colored mini-lights around inside bedroom windows, doors or along ceiling.

☐Insert notes and letters, photos, or small magnetic calendars in Christmas cards.

☐Listen to recorded Christmas music.

☐Make a Christmas banner by gluing felt pieces — Nativity figures, stars, Christmas trees, or other simple holiday patterns, on a large, rectangular piece of felt.

❑Make a Christmas ornament from a craft kit.

❑Make a simple Christmas pin to give as a gift or wear on your collar.

❑Make Christmas candy.

❑Make gift wrap paper. **Caregiver**: Use white or other solid-color paper and have your AD family member decorate it with stencils, water color paints, felt-tipped pens, colored pencils, stamps, or holiday pictures cut from magazines. Apply white paint to solid blue paper to create falling snow, snowy hillsides, and snowmen. Snowflake shapes cut from white paper and glued on a blue background are also lovely. Add silver glitter for extra pizazz.

❑Place postal stamps and decorative stamps on envelopes.

"We had assumed Gramps remembered how to put postal stamps on envelopes, but he didn't. After we discovered several stamps on wrong corners, we showed him how to do it and he did a great job after that."

❑Put a Christmas tablecloth on the table.

❑Put bows and ribbon on packages.

❑Put Christmas cards in envelopes and seal.

❑Put candy or cookies in small, decorative bags for gift-giving.

❐Put candles in candleholders.

❐Set up Nativity figures.

❐Shop for gifts.

❐Sign greeting cards, or affix your signature with a rubber stamp.

❐Sort candles by colors.

❐Stroll through a mall and look at Christmas decorations.

❐Talk about past family Christmases. What is your happiest Christmas memory? How did your family celebrate Christmas when you were a child? What kind of decorations did you put on your Christmas tree? What favorite foods did you eat at Christmas? Did relatives come to visit or did you visit them? What was the best gift you ever received?

❐Visit a Christmas tree farm.

❐Visit a toy store and discuss childhood memories of Christmases and toys.

❐Visit the Christmas section at a department store.

❐Walk through your neighborhood to look at Christmas decorations. If it's not too cold, take your walk after dark when lights will be on.

❐Watch a Christmas video classic — *It's a Wonderful Life, Frosty the Snowman, Santa Claus Is Coming to Town, Rudolph the Red-nosed Reindeer, The Nutcracker,* and others.

☐Wear a variety of Christmas pins and other
holiday jewelry during December.
☐Wrap gifts.

Cinco de Mayo (May 5)

On May 5, 1862, untrained and outnumbered Mexican guerilla forces successfully defended the strategic town of Puebla against French troops. Filled with hope and courage, Mexicans committed themselves to the cause of national hero Benito Juárez, which eventually led to the end of European domination. Cinco de Mayo symbolizes the right of people to self-determination and national sovereignty and is celebrated in Mexican-American communities throughout the United States.

☐Attend mass.
☐Attend a school or public program of Mexican
music and dancing.
☐Bake traditional cookies or pastry.
☐Call a friend and tell him you're proud of him.
☐Decorate a room with the Mexican flag or
colors.
☐Eat dinner in a Mexican restaurant.
☐Listen to Mexican music.
☐Read a story about a famous Mexican.
☐Share your family memorabilia, scrapbooks, or
photo albums with a child.
☐Make a traditional Mexican dessert for dinner.
☐Play a Mexican game.

☐Talk about your Mexican-American heritage. When did you or your ancestors arrive in the United States? How did they get here? Where did they live. What type work did they do? What was the best thing they experienced? What was the most difficult?

The Civil War (1861-1865)

This war occurred more than 135 years ago when President Abraham Lincoln was in office so no one living today will remember it. However, military history buffs and some old-timers have wonderful stories to share about men who fought in the Civil War and family members whose lives were changed as a result of it.

☐Browse through a Civil War picture book.
☐Read a book or story about the Civil War, perhaps a children's book from the library.
☐Subscribe to a magazine featuring historical information and photos of the Civil War — *America's Civil War, American Heritage,* or others.
☐Talk about famous men and women who lived during the Civil War — Abraham Lincoln, Ulysses S. Grant, Robert E. Lee, Thomas J. "Stonewall" Jackson, William T. Sherman or others. Did you learn about any of these people in school? Why do you think they were important?

☐Talk about your family's memories and stories of the Civil War. In what states did your ancestors live during the Civil War? Did men in your family fight in battles?

☐Tell Civil War stories — true or fictional — you have heard or read.

☐Tour a Civil War battle site.

☐Visit a Civil War memorial or museum.

"Ezra grew up in Alabama and recalls with a chuckle that when he was a boy, two old Civil War veterans — one from the North and one from the South — used to get into arguments about the war and hit each other with their canes."

"Fiona treasures family letters written by her great-grandfather to his wife and children during the Civil War. The last letter was written just before he died in Andersonville Military Prison in Georgia."

Confederate States, 1861

Alabama, Florida, Virginia, North Carolina, South Carolina, Georgia, Tennessee, Arkansas, Mississippi, Louisiana, Texas

Union States, 1861

California, Oregon, Maine, Vermont, New Hampshire, Massachusetts, Connecticut, Rhode Island, New Jersey, New York, Pennsylvania, Ohio, Indiana, Illinois, Michigan, Wisconsin, Minnesota, Iowa, Kansas

---

Clothing

From the time we are young children, clothes play an important part in our lives. We take pride in learning to button, zip, tie shoelaces, put on shirts, pants, boots, hats and sweaters. For years we routinely perform these tasks, and then one day, when Alzheimer's disease begins to take its toll, these and other activities of daily life become challenges. Encourage your AD family member to do what he or she can, even if it takes a long time. Be patient and resist the urge to help out too soon.

☐Button shirts, blouses and sweaters.
☐Check garments for loose buttons.
☐Fold handkerchiefs.
☐Go to a fashion show.
☐Shop for clothes. **Caregiver**: It may be less confusing and stressful to shop for only one item — a pair of shoes or a sweater.
☐Hand-wash lingerie or socks.
☐Hang clothes in the closet.
☐Iron clothes. **Caregiver**: Allow this task only if your AD family member can do it safely.
☐Organize shoes or boots in the closet.
☐Polish or shine shoes.
☐Put clean clothing in drawers.
☐Put dirty clothing in the laundry hamper.
☐Tie shoelaces.

> *"When Claudine lived alone, she wore dirty, ragged outfits all the time. After she*

*was diagnosed with Alzheimer's disease,
she moved in with her niece, who bought
Claudine new clothes and helped her
clean up. Claudine smiles a lot more now
and says she feels pretty."*

Collections

*There's no limit to the number of interesting items that
can be enjoyably collected, looked at, sorted, and shared.
If your AD family member does not already have a collection, consider beginning one. Limit the collection to
small items — buttons, postcards, rings, dolls, tiny perfume bottles, miniature figures, fountain pens, pocket
watches, sports trading cards, stamps, or others.*

☐ Add a new item to your collection every month
  or two.
☐ Decorate a sturdy cardboard box in which to
  store your collection.
☐ Display your special collection in a glass case
  or on a shelf or tabletop.
☐ Invite a friend to share and tell you about his or
  her collection.
☐ Make a list of the items in your collection. How
  many do you have?
☐ Share your collection and stories about the
  items with a friend or group.
☐ Talk about collections you have seen or heard
  about. What was the most unusual collection?

The largest collection? Most expensive? Most fun?

❏ Talk about your collection. Where did you get the items? How long did it take you to collect them? Why did you decide to collect them?

❏ Visit a museum to look at other collections.

Columbus Day
(Second Monday in October, formerly October 12)

This holiday honors Christopher Columbus' discovery of America on October 12, 1492. Columbus was not the first explorer to arrive in the Western Hemisphere, but his exploration opened the way for settlement of America by Europeans.

❏ Attend local parades and celebrations.

❏ Call Italian friends and wish them a happy Columbus Day.

❏ Color or paint pictures of Columbus or his ships — the Nina, the Pinta and the Santa Maria.

❏ Help prepare food.

    ❏ Arrange cheese and salami on a plate.

    ❏ Fill pasta pans with cold water.

    ❏ Pour croutons into salad.

    ❏ Pour dry pasta into measuring cups.

    ❏ Place bread sticks in a glass.

    ❏ Put olives in a bowl.

    ❏ Scoop spumoni ice cream into small bowls and decorate with sprinkles and maraschino cherries.

☐Slice cheese.

☐Spread garlic butter on bread.

☐Sprinkle parmesan cheese on pasta, salad or soup.

☐Stir pasta sauce.

☐Tear up lettuce for salad.

☐Toss salad.

☐Wash and cut up vegetables for ministrone soup.

☐Decorate with preprinted or hand-drawn cutouts of the Nina, the Pinta and the Santa Maria, Columbus, Italian flags, or a map of Italy.

☐Drink Italian coffee or wine (Nonalcoholic wine is available.) served with biscotti.

☐Eat out at a pizza parlor or Italian restaurant.

☐Eat spumoni ice cream for dessert.

☐Fly an Italian flag.

☐Listen to Italian music — modern or opera. **Caregiver**: Check your library for rentals.

☐On a globe, examine Columbus' route to the New World.

☐Put small, paper Italian flags at place settings.

☐Sing an Italian song — *That's Amore* ("When the moon hits your eye like a big pizza pie, that's amore ..."), *Funniculi, Funnicula, Arrivederci Roma*, and others.

☐Talk about well-known or famous Italians in your community or the world.

☐Visit the library and read a short book or story about Columbus.

☐Watch a video about Columbus. **Caregiver**: Check your local video store or library for rentals.

Computers

Even if your AD family member or patient has little or no computer experience, he or she may enjoy some of the simple games and activities designed for children. If typing is still an option, writing e-mail notes or letters may be pleasurable, or have the patient "dictate" what he or she wants to say while you type.

❑Borrow and experiment with a simple computer activity from the library.

❑Enjoy e-mail letters. **Caregiver**: Create your own letters from favorite distant relatives if they don't correspond often, or save old e-mail letters and reread them from time to time.

❑Play the interactive CD-ROM computer game *Road Construction Ahead.* **Caregiver**: Ideal for men, the player uses heavy equipment to dig, blast and build his own roads. (Fred Levine Productions).

Crafts

Simple craft projects can be finished relatively quickly or worked on daily for a longer period of time. Select projects that will appeal to your AD family member or patient's interests and are appropriate for skill level.

❑Create colorful candles. **Caregiver**: Kits, molds and how-to books are available at craft stores.

☐Create a colorful flower garden or pastoral landscape on paper. **Caregiver**: Help your AD family member cut pictures from calendars, greeting cards, seed catalogs and magazines to create a scene on a piece of construction paper. (Solid, light blue paper or a blue painted sky make good backgrounds.) Then, using a glue stick, combine favorite flowers. For dimension, attach small, double-stick foam blocks to a few flowers and glue stretched cotton-ball clouds in the sky.

☐Decorate canvas shoes with painted designs.

☐Discuss favorite things, then find examples of them in magazines. **Caregiver**: Help cut out pictures, paste them on a piece of construction paper, and label each. (e.g., kittens, pink flowers, hugs, pretty quilts)

☐Enjoy a lacing kit. **Caregiver**: Buy a kit that has a ready-cut project, safety needles and yarn. Kits are available through craft stores, catalogs, and Elder Press.

☐Make refrigerator magnets. **Caregiver**: Use felt designs or small objects and purchased magnets that can be glued on.

☐Make soap. **Caregiver**: Kits, molds and how-to books are available at craft stores.

☐Press flowers and leaves. **Caregiver**: Glue the pressed flowers and leaves on note cards or stationery and seal by laminating.

☐String beads.

Dance Marathons

If your patient is 65 years or older, he or she may remember dance marathons, which were "all the rage" during the 1920s and well into the 1930s. The fun began on March 31, 1923, when Alma Cummings set a world record of 27 hours of continuous dancing.

❏Dance with someone who remembers the 1920s and 1930s. **Caregiver**: Play music of the era for a perfect mood.

❏Look at photographs taken during the 1920s and 1930s.

❏Reminisce about everyday life during the 1920s and 1930s. How old were you during that era? What entertainments did you enjoy? Did you ever participate in a dance marathon? What was it like?

❏Teach someone a dance step from the 1920s or 1930s.

❏Watch a movie musical set in the 1920s or 1930s.

Day Care Programs

The best thing I ever did for my father and for me was to enroll him in the Primrose Alzheimer's Day Club a couple times a week. He thrives on the attention and activities, and I get a much-needed break from our usual routine. To ease possible stress during your AD family member's transition from home care to organized day care, refer to the program as a "day club," "adult exercise program," "senior citizen center," or other title that will be received positively.

☐Describe what you ate at breakfast, lunch, dinner and/or snack times. **Caregiver**: If daily menus are not posted, ask the day care director what was served and what your family member ate, because he or she may not remember later. This information is important for nutritional reasons and to help you communicate about the day's events.

> *"I worried when Minnie told me the only thing she'd had to eat all day was the cookie she was eating when I arrived to pick her up. As it turned out she'd eaten three meals that she had forgotten."*

☐Share a favorite activity with friends in your day activity program. **Caregiver**: Encourage your family member to take games, puzzles, or other activities enjoyed at home to share with day club friends. Home craft projects and art work can also be displayed at day club.

☐Talk about activities you enjoy. **Caregiver**: Quality day care programs post daily activities schedules for the week or month. In addition, your family member will have free time to take leisurely walks in the secure environment, visit or play games with friends, read, watch television, or snooze in a comfortable chair. Review the schedule each day and ask the day care director which activities your family member participated in and enjoyed. Feel free to recommend additional activities. Activity directors are always looking for new ideas.

> *"My husband, Jack, did not want to join the Alzheimer's day care program until I told him his doctor had ordered it for the exercise benefits. Once Jack tried it, he liked it very much."*

Dolls

Many women continue their childhood love of dolls and cuddly toys throughout their lifetime. Providing a "lovey" for your AD family member may help reassure and calm her, especially during stressful periods.

☐Browse through a book about dolls, especially a pictorial history.

☐Collect and display miniature dolls.

☐Comb and arrange dolls' hair.

☐Cuddle dolls and soft stuffed animals.

☐Dress dolls. **Caregiver**: If buttons and snaps are difficult, glue or sew on Velcro strips, or fashion loose fitting garments that only need to be slipped over the doll's head.

☐Keep a scrapbook of doll pictures cut from magazines and catalogs.

☐Knit doll blankets.

☐Play "dolls" with a child.

☐Read a story about a doll — Raggedy Ann, Patty Reed's Doll (a doll's eye view of the pioneering Donner Party's journey from Illinois to California), or others.

☐Look at doll collector magazines. Subscriptions are generally pricey, so compare offers before you order, and look for doll magazines at your local library and thrift stores, too.

☐Talk about childhood dolls and doll playing experiences. How many dolls did you have? Did you collect dolls? Did your mother or grandmother make you a rag doll? What dolls were popular when you were growing up — Bye-lo Baby, Dionne Quintuplets, Shirley Temple? Did you have a doll house?

☐Tell about your favorite childhood doll. What was her name? What did she look like? Was she a large doll or a small doll? A big girl or a baby? Did she have "real" hair? Eyes that opened and closed? Could you feed her a bottle and change her diaper? Who gave your favorite doll to you, or where did you get her? How old were you? Did you play dolls with friends? What were their names?

☐Wash hands and faces of vinyl dolls.

☐Wear a miniature doll pin.

Easter (Date varies)

Easter falls on the first Sunday after the first full moon following March 21, the vernal equinox, which is the day in spring when day and night are of equal length.

Easter, the most important Christian holy day, celebrates the resurrection of Jesus Christ on the third day after his sacrificial crucifixion to save people from their sins.

Easter has also evolved as a traditional nonreligious American holiday, celebrating springtime with family gatherings, egg decorating, baskets filled with eggs and candy, egg hunts, stories about the Easter bunny, new clothes, and gifts of toy bunnies, chicks and lambs. Easter is believed to have taken its name from the Teutonic festival of Eostur, celebrating spring's return each year.

☐Attend church services.

☐Attend an Easter sunrise service.

☐Bake and decorate a cross-, rabbit-, or egg-shaped cake. **Caregiver**: Buy specialty cake pans in cake-decorating departments and stores.

☐Bake and decorate Easter cookies.

☐Call friends and wish them happy Easter.

☐Coat a canned ham with seasoned sauce or add pineapple and cloves before cooking.

☐Create spring floral arrangements.

☐Decorate boiled eggs with egg-coloring kits.

☐Decorate blown egg shells with felt-tipped pens, acrylic paints, colorful stickers, or by marbelizing with paint.

❑Don an Easter bonnet.

❑Fill an Easter basket for a child.

❑Listen to spiritual music celebrating Christ's resurrection.

❑Look at family Easter photographs.

❑Purchase or hand-craft Easter decorations on stakes to place in lawn and along walkways.

❑Read a children's story about Christ's death and resurrection.

❑Read a biblical account of Christ's death and resurrection.

❑Send an Easter card to someone.

❑Stuff a giant plastic or cloth rabbit to sit on your front porch.

❑Stuff deviled eggs, sprinkle them with paprika, and decorate with parsley sprigs.

❑Talk about bygone Easter experiences. What is your first Easter memory? What was your happiest Easter? What did you like best about Easter? Did you go to church on Easter Sunday? Did you get new clothes for Easter? Did you decorate and hunt for Easter eggs?

❑Wear an Easter pin.

"Every now and then go away, have a little relaxation, for when you come back to your work your judgment will be surer. . . . "
—Leonardo Da Vinci

Ecology

Biological ecology focuses on the interrelationship of animals, including mankind, and the environment. You can help make the world a better place with earth-nurturing activities.

☐Collect and crush aluminum cans for recycling.
☐Collect recyclable plastic containers for recycling.
☐Create a bird and butterfly garden. **Caregiver:** How-to books listing plants that nurture birds and butterflies are available at book stores, libraries and through the internet.
☐Fill bird feeders.
☐Gather flower seeds after blooming season.
☐Handcraft paper from a kit.
☐Plant a seedling tree.
☐Plant flowers.
☐Raise earthworms. **Caregiver:** It's really easy and a great way to dispose of vegetable waste from your kitchen. In return, the worms give you premium soil. You'll find information on raising worms at libraries, bookstores and through the Internet.
☐Sow wildflower seeds.
☐Start a compost pile for kitchen and other vegetable waste. **Caregiver:** Check out the above resources for how-to information.
☐Tie newspapers and magazines into bundles for recycling.

Election Day

In 1845 Congress established the first Tuesday after the first Monday in November as General Election Day. The President and Vice-President are elected in those years evenly divisible by four. On even years, members of the House of Representatives are elected for two-year terms and one-third of the Senate for six-year terms. Every November, there are elections somewhere in the United States. Special local elections may occur at other times.

(See politics section for activities.)

Exercise

Exercise is important for all people, including those with impaired memories. Significant, regular movement helps keep muscles toned and bowel movements regular. Some caregivers report that exercise also decreases their loved ones' agitation and restlessness and helps them sleep better at night. Caregivers should remember to exercise regularly, too, for all of the above reasons. Consult a physician before beginning any exercise program.

❒Bat a balloon to a partner.
❒Bounce or play catch with a ball. **Caregiver**: Select the ball's size and weight to accommodate your AD family member's skill level.
❒Dance.
❒Lift light weights. **Caregiver**: If you don't have dumbbells, try unbreakable plastic containers

— small water or soda bottle, or other container that is easy to hold.

☐ Stroll in an enclosed shopping mall during less-than-ideal weather.

☐ Walk, even a short distance, every day if possible.

☐ Watch and follow along to easy-to-do exercise videos or televised exercise programs.

☐ Strengthen and tone specific parts of the body using rubberized stretch bands.

"While recovering from a broken arm, Mother resisted exercising unless I joined her. When I did, she smiled and worked out like a trooper. In the long run, we both benefitted."

"My Dad's physical therapist recommended that both he and I use stretch bands to strengthen our arms and legs and improve our posture. I bought a set of inexpensive bands at her office, and she gave us an illustrated pamphlet showing how Dad could do the exercises sitting down and I, standing up. It was fun and easy."

"The sovereign invigorator of the body is exercise, and of all the exercises walking is best."
—Thomas Jefferson, 1786

Family History

Who we are, where we came from, and what we've experienced is important and should be appreciated and respected.

☐ Buy a special frame to hold a favorite family photograph.

☐ Have a family group photo taken.

☐ Keep a journal of family experiences you remember. **Caregiver**: If your AD family member needs help, write recollections in the journal as they are recalled and read them back to him or her later.

☐ Share a family story with a relative, perhaps a child, and answer questions.

☐ Sort through family photographs. **Caregiver**: Document names, places and dates.

☐ Talk about your family experiences. **Caregiver**: Write or record with audio- or videotape family stories and anecdotal information.

☐ Tape record the story of a family experience to give to a relative. Ask him or her to tape a remembered experience for you.

☐ Visit the library, or perhaps a genealogical resource center, and read the history of your surname.

"It seems so strange that my mother can no longer remember who I am, but she can still name her cousins and schoolmates in old childhood photos."

Farms/Ranches

Until the 1920s, most Americans lived in rural areas, and long after that time, many continued to live or work on farms and ranches. If your AD family member or patient was fortunate enough to have had this experience, or simply dreamed of it, he or she will probably enjoy some of the following activities.

☐Bottle feed an orphaned calf, goat or lamb.

☐Browse through a picture book on farm or ranch history.

☐Collect postcards of farm and ranch scenes.

☐Create a barnyard or ranch collage. **Caregiver**: Help your family member find and cut favorite pictures from country magazines or calendars. Glue them onto construction paper.

☐Enjoy a hayride.

☐Feast on old-fashioned farm food — fried chicken, mashed potatoes and gravy, corn on the cob, biscuits, berry cobbler.

☐Feed apples or carrots to horses or goats.

☐Gather eggs.

☐Go to a country fair and tour the livestock and poultry barns. What is your favorite animal? Were you a member of 4-H (a farming club for young people sponsored by the U.S. Department of Agriculture) or FFA (Future Farmers of America) when you were growing up? Did you ever raise animals to show or sell at a fair? What kind? Did they win ribbons?

Was raising animals hard work? How did you care for your animals?

☐Have your picture taken on the farm and mail a copy to a friend.

☐Look at family snapshots taken on the farm. Identify people, places and dates and write the information on photo backs with acid-free permanent ink.

☐Make a scrapbook of farm or ranch pictures cut from magazines.

☐Read a story about farm life.

☐Sample fresh fruit from an orchard or vineyard.

☐Subscribe to a magazine that features farm life — *Country*, *Country Woman*, *Country Journal*.

☐Take a ride through the country during springtime when trees are in blossom and newborn animals graze in pastures, or in the fall when leaves turn color.

☐Talk about living, working or vacationing on a farm or ranch. When did you do that? What did you like best about farm or ranch life? What did you like least? What time did you get up in the morning? How has farming changed? What are your favorite farm animals?

☐Ride in a horse-drawn carriage or wagon.

☐Scatter grain to free-range chickens, ducks or other fowl.

☐Tour a museum or display of antique farm equipment.

☐Tour a working farm or ranch.
☐Visit a farm that raises prized or unusual stock and offers tours — cattle, game birds, horses, llamas, ponies, potbellied pigs, pygmy goats, miniature horses, and others.
☐Wear a straw hat, a colorful bandana around your neck and, if you have them, cowboy boots.

> *"When I was a little girl, I often tagged along with Daddy while he milked cows, plowed fields, and mended fences."*

Father's Day
(Third Sunday in June)

In 1910, the first Father's Day was celebrated in Spokane, Washington. The holiday became official in 1924 when President Calvin Coolidge proclaimed the third Sunday in June as Father's Day. Roses are the flowers of the day: red to be worn if your father is living; white if your father is dead.

☐Arrange a bouquet of roses as a centerpiece.
☐Bake or decorate a Father's Day cake for a special man. **Caregiver**: On a sheet cake, outline a collar and necktie to fill in with color, designs or sprinkles.
☐Call a young father and wish him a happy Father's Day.

❑Look at photographs of your father.
❑Talk about your father. What did he look like? How tall was he? Do you look like him? What was his personality like? Is your personality like his? Did you have the same interests? What did you like best about your father? What did you like least . . . or dislike?
❑Walk through a rose garden.
❑Wear a corsage of roses or a boutonniere in honor of your father or because you are a father.

Field Trips

Possibilities for field trips are limitless. Select those that appeal to your AD family member and you, nothing too time-consuming or strenuous. Take along a camera to capture the fun, and snacks or drinks if your adventure will not be near food vendors.

> **NOTE:** Before feeding animals in public places, check with authorities or posted signs for rules and regulations.

❑Break up stale bread and put it in bags to feed to fish and fowl.
❑Discover birds . . . with binoculars or the naked eye. Join a bird-watching group on a short, easy walk.
❑Enjoy the excitement of an auto race.

☐Feed ducks at the lake, pigeons in the park, or sea gulls at the seashore.

☐Go to an air show.

☐Recapture childhood thrills at a circus.

☐Relax at a movie matinee. Eat popcorn.

☐Schedule a few hours at a country fair. **Caregiver**: Many offer discounted entrance prices for senior citizens and physically challenged people, and free rides for all around the fairgrounds. Buy cotton candy or a snow cone. Visit buildings that display cooking, sewing, and woodworking projects, cake decorating, art, photography and livestock.

☐Sit in an airport terminal or in a car near the airport and watch planes take off and land.

☐Spend some time at a dog park and watch them romp, retrieve balls, and catch Frisbees.

☐Stroll along a level, tree-lined street during blossom time or when leaves change color in the fall.

☐Tour a fish hatchery and feed fingerlings.

☐Tour a museum.

☐Visit an art gallery or business establishment that displays the work of local artists. Discuss favorite works and why they are appealing.

☐Using photos taken on a fieldtrip, along with souvenirs, make a scrapbook of the event. Record names, date, and place.

☐Visit a local flower nursery that offers special attractions such as fish ponds, waterfalls, picnic tables under shady trees, lanes for strolling, floral displays.

❏ Watch a sunset while nibbling on cookies and iced tea, or a sunrise while sipping a hot beverage and pastry.

Fishing

Some people fish for their livelihoods while others fish for pleasure. Whichever, fish stories usually originate in youth and remain vivid into old age. If you are caring for a fisherman or fisherwoman, you will find abundant fun things to do and talk about.

❏ Collect fishing gear — lures, poles, creels.

❏ Collect miniature fishing boats.

❏ Collect pictures and postcards of fishing scenes.

❏ Create a fishing collage with pictures cut from fishing magazines, or use fish stickers available at craft stores.

❏ Enjoy a seafood dinner.

❏ Go to a nearby pond, lake or river to fish.
   Caregiver: If your family member uses a walker or wheelchair, or is unsteady on his or her feet, make sure the fishing area is accessible and safe.

❏ Hang a fish mobile from the ceiling.

❏ Play a mechanical fishing game in which the fish move around the game tray, their mouths opening and closing regularly. **Caregiver**: Each player holds a miniature fishing pole with a magnet on the end of the line and catches fish by dropping the magnet into its metal-lined mouth. There are several variations of this game available in different sizes. I prefer the larger size (under $10) from Pressman, available at Wal-Mart and elsewhere.

☐Play the card game *Go Fish/Fish*.

☐Put your picture in a frame decorated with a fishing theme.

☐Raise earthworms for bait. (*See ecology section for how-to information.*)

☐Share fish stories. When did you learn to fish? Who taught you? What was the biggest fish you ever caught? What type bait did you use? Where was the best fishing? Who were your fishing partners?

☐Subscribe to a fishing magazine. **Caregiver**: Set aside a regular time to look at, read and discuss topics in the magazine.

☐Talk about fish you caught — bass, bullheads, carp, catfish, cod, crappies, bluegill, eel, flounder, halibut, perch, pickerel, pike, rockfish, salmon, sunfish, steelhead, sturgeon, trout, tuna or others. Which were your favorite to catch and to eat? How were they cooked?

☐Talk about fishing bait you used — cheese, crayfish pieces, grasshoppers, minnows, pork chunks or rinds, salmon eggs, small pieces of fish, worms or others.

☐ Talk about fishing boats you owned or enjoyed — commercial, rowboat, motorboat, sailboat or other. When did you get your first boat? How many boats have you owned? On what bodies of water — bays, lakes, rivers, oceans — did you fish from your boat? What type vehicle did you use to pull your boat?

☐ Talk about fishing lures you used — dry or streamer flies or nymphs (for fly fishing), wobblers, plugs, spinners (for bait fishing), or others.

☐ Talk about shellfish or mollusks you dug, trapped, netted or captured by other means — abalone, clam, crab, lobster, octopus, oyster, shrimp, squid or others.

☐ Talk about the type of fishing rod and reel you used — fly, spinning, bait-casting or other. Why was this a good rod for you? When you were a child did you ever fish with a pole cut from cane, bamboo, or a willow branch? Was that fun? Did you use a commercial hook or make one? What bait did you use? What type fish did you catch?

☐ Visit a fish hatchery.

☐ Visit a fishing supplies store and look at classic and new equipment. Talk about the different products. Which items (fishing rods, lures, tackle boxes, etc.) do you like best? How much did these things cost in years gone by?

What is your favorite fishing memory? How has fishing changed during your lifetime?

Flag Day (June 14)

This holiday is the anniversary of the day Congress adopted the stars and stripes as the national emblem of the United States, June 14, 1777.

☐Discuss the United States flag's design. What colors is it? (*red, white and blue*) What is the design? (*stars and stripes*) Do you know what the stars and stripes represent? (*The stripes represent the original 13 colonies that rebelled against England. The stars represent the states in the union.*)

☐Decorate a flag cake. Spread white frosting, whipped cream, or nondairy topping on a sheet cake, add blueberries for stars and rows of sliced strawberries for stripes.

☐Draw or paint a picture of the U.S. flag.

☐Guess how many times the U.S. flag has changed since it was adopted in 1777. (*The answer is 26, each time a new state joined the union.*) Since 1818, the only change has been the addition of new stars.

☐List the original thirteen colonies. **Caregiver**: Make a game of how many can be remembered. Give liberal hints, and reward each right or near-right answer with a special treat

— a piece of wrapped candy or other. For a group of patients in an AD facility, give a prize to those born or having lived in states that were part of the original thirteen colonies.

America's Thirteen Original Colonies	
Connecticut	New York
Delaware	North Carolina
Georgia	Pennsylvania
Maryland	Rhode Island
Massachusetts	South Carolina
New Hampshire	Virginia
New Jersey	

❑Look through a picture book showing the history of the United States flag. How has it changed through the years? Which flag do you like best?

❑Make a red, white and blue gelatin dessert.

❑Place gold stars on a map showing the location of each of the original 13 colonies. **Caregiver**: Make this easier by marking an X or drawing a small star where each gold star should be placed.

❑Put up, take down and fold the flag.

❑Read or listen to the words of Francis Scott Key's song *The Star Spangled Banner*. What do the words mean to you?

❑Talk about the stars in the U.S. flag. Do you remember when the U.S. flag had fewer stars than it has now? What states have joined the union during your lifetime?

❑Visit the library and look through a book picturing flags of the world. Which flags do you like best? Have you ever seen a flag from another country? Which one? When and where did you see it? Did your family have a flag from the country they or your ancestors came from? What colors was it? Did it have stripes or a symbol on it? What did the symbol stand for?
❑Wear a flag pin on your collar.

Foods & Beverages

The clock of life ticks to the rhythm of daily meals, family gatherings and special occasions where favorite foods and beverages are served.

❑Choose favorite foods and beverages for mealtimes and snacks. **Caregiver**: List favorite foods on a sheet of paper or duplicate an extensive list from which your family member can make selections each day or week. Choices should result in balanced meals.
❑Dip freshly cut fruit in lemon juice or other preservative to keep it from turning brown.
❑Drink eight glasses of water daily. **Caregiver**: Water is beneficial to health, and most of us don't drink enough. Encourage water consumption by placing a measured quantity in an attractive glass container and making a game of regularly drinking a glassful.

☐Eat "comfort foods" once in a while. **Caregiver**: These favorites remind us of special times and special people and help us feel relaxed and emotionally secure. Unfortunately, the comfort foods we generally prefer are loaded with fat: Grandma's fried chicken, buttery biscuits, bacon gravy, whipped cream cake, chocolate, doughnuts, potato chips, and other fatty delights. To maintain good health, save comfort foods for special occasions only.

☐Enjoy meals and snacks. **Caregiver**: This sounds easy, but it can be challenging. Success is largely dependent on the caregiver's planning and attitude. Maintain a regular dining/snack schedule, prepare easy-to-eat foods, and relax as much as possible. Smile, communicate gently and, above all, be as patient as an angel.

☐Make a collage of favorite foods. **Caregiver**: Help cut pictures from magazines and paste them on construction paper.

☐Try a new food or beverage. **Caregiver**: Many healthy products are available, including snack foods and fruit juice combinations. Check out health foods and standard products at grocery stores. Read labels for nutrition information. (I recently discovered barbecue-flavored rice cakes. Fantastic!)

Caregiver: Remember to take care of yourself.

Food Preparation

Food preparation is one of the most meaningful activities in life. It provides an opportunity to show off skills and talents, and results in nourishment for the body and soul . . . and compliments!

> **Note: Be sure to give step-by-step instructions, one step at a time, and be specific.**

> *"Magda was told she could crack the eggs on the table, so she cracked them, opened them up, and poured the yolks on the table instead of in the bowl."*

☐Add nuts, chocolate chips, etc. to batter.

☐Arrange cooled cookies on a plate.

☐Bag and freeze fresh, in-season blueberries.
Caregiver: Do not wash blueberries until you use them. (The grayish coating helps to preserve them.) Simply put blueberries in small freezer bags, seal or close with a twisty-tie, and freeze.

☐Beat eggs.

☐Cut out cookies with cookie cutters.

☐Cut vegetables or fruit.

☐Crack eggs for a recipe.

☐Decorate cookies and cakes.

☐Drain liquid from canned food products — fruit, olives, beets, etc.

☐Fill and seal cookies.

☐Fill sugar and creamer bowls.
☐Fill water glasses at mealtime.
☐Fill and seal won-ton wrappers.
☐Grate carrots.
☐Grate cheese.
☐Grease cookie sheets or cake pans.
☐Help bake, adding one ingredient at a time.
☐Knead bread dough.
☐Make butter curls.
☐Make candy. Candy recipes that do not
    require cooking are especially easy.
☐Peel hard boiled eggs.
☐Peel potatoes or other vegetables and fruit.
☐Put toppings on cookies, cakes, ice cream
    sundaes or puddings.
☐Remove biscuits from a pressurized can,
    separate them, and arrange them on a baking
    sheet.
☐Roll cookie or pie dough with a rolling pin.
☐Shape hamburger into patties.
☐Shred lettuce.
☐Slice cookie dough from a pressurized can and
    arrange on baking sheet.
☐Slice bar cookies.
☐Spoon cookie dough onto a baking tray.
☐Squeeze lemon or orange juice using a
    hand-juicer.
☐Stir batter.
☐Wash fruit and vegetables.
☐Whip cream.

Fragrances and Scents

A fragrance is a pleasant thing, but it can be more. In the time it takes to inhale the scent of a flower, perfume or pipe tobacco, we may be mentally transported back in time to an experience in which that same scent was present. In memory, we relive the event's action and emotion. Take advantage of these opportunities for better communication with your AD family member and patients.

☐Make sachets. **Caregiver**: Dry (or buy dried) flower petals (roses or lavender) and add perfumed oils to fill lingerie drawer sachets.

☐Purchase perfumed sachets to put in lingerie drawers.

☐Reminisce about the fragrances of your mother, father, grandparents or babies.

☐Stroll through a fragrant garden. Take time to stop and smell the flowers.

☐Sniff samples of fragrant wood — cedar, balsam, redwood, pine.

☐Talk about your favorite and your least favorite fragrances and odors. What was the best thing you ever smelled? The worst thing? What is your favorite food fragrance? What is your favorite perfume or after shave?

☐Use favorite perfume, talcum powder or after-shave.

☐Visit a department store cosmetic department and sample perfumes.

"Lavender sachets make Mary Lynn happy, reminding her of her mother and grandmother, who always kept sachets in their bureau drawers."

"Van says the odor of a certain disinfectant sends him back to his childhood and the hospital where he had his tonsils removed."

Games
(Fine Motor & Mental)

Games stimulate the brain and help maintain or improve eye-hand coordination. Numerous easy games are offered through retail outlets and online. You may also find appropriate children's games in your closets or at yard sales. If one game doesn't work for your AD family member, try another. An alternative for difficult games is to include the AD patient as the tile shuffler, dice roller or timekeeper who lets players know when the timer rings.

☐Delight in *Dominoes*. **Caregiver**: Use two sets to make the game easier. Be flexible with rules, helping your AD family member succeed on individual plays and win games. Enjoy dominoes in other ways, too. Stack colored dominoes by colors, build simple structures, or stand a row of tiles on end and send them tumbling with a flick of your finger.

☐Discover CD-ROM *Memory Works Matching games*. **Caregiver**: These games were developed by the Practical Memory Institute (PMI) and are available online through MemoryZine.

☐Draw or write with *Etch-a-Sketch*.

☐Enjoy *Around-the-Home Lotto*. **Caregiver**: A set of 72-picture cards, $14.95, is available through Super Duper Publications.

☐*Finish the Proverb*. **Caregiver**: This verbal game can be played at home, in the car, or while waiting at the doctor's office. You recite the beginning of a proverb, and your AD family member finishes it. *A bird in the hand . . . is worth two in the bush. You never miss the water . . . 'til the well runs dry. A penny saved . . . is a penny earned. April showers . . . bring May flowers. Haste . . . makes waste. A stitch in time . . . saves nine.*

☐Go fishing with a mechanical *fishing game*. **Caregiver**: This small wind-up toy has fishing poles with magnetized "hooks" to catch rotating fish whose magnetized mouths open and shut for a simple challenge. Available at retail stores and through Pressman Corporation.

☐Have a sweet time with *Candyland*.

☐Play with *Pla-Doh* and Pla-Doh molds. **Caregiver**: Price varies depending on the size of the set. I recommend starting with a small set.

☐Plug into *Pegboards*. **Caregiver**: Pegboards

with easy grip pegs are perfect for rigid fingers. Under $25. Elder Press.
☐Recall childhood with an *Uncle Wiggly* board game.
☐Relax with *Bingo*. **Caregiver**: There are many varieties of bingo at varying prices. Compare them at educational, variety and toy stores, online, and through Super Duper Publications.
☐Say yes to *Yahtzee*.

Games (Large Muscle)

The following games have been successfully played as family activities. Revise rules, adapting them as the game progresses, if necessary. The outcome should be a winning situation for your AD family member.

☐Balance or bounce a tennis ball on a racket.
☐Bounce a basketball.
☐Bowl at public bowling lanes or, with a small ball and pins, on the lawn or in the family room. **Caregiver**: Even if your family member is not able to participate, consider taking him or her along to watch others bowl, kibitz, and offer bowling tips.
☐Enjoy miniature golf. Play on public courses or buy home sets for lawn or indoor use.
☐Hit a tennis ball with a racket.
☐Pitch horseshoes.
☐Play catch with a beach ball or softball.

☐Play catch with a Velcro paddle and ball.

☐Play bocce ball.

☐Relax with lawn croquet.

☐Shine on the shuffleboard court.

☐Throw a beanbag. **Caregiver**: A beanbag can be tossed from one person to another or at a target. **To make a beanbag**, cut sturdy scrap fabric in any shape desired. Double-stitch around the edges, leaving a small opening for filling. Turn inside out, fill with dried beans, and double-stitch the hole closed. **To make a target**, use a large piece of plywood or heavy cardboard, cut one or more holes in it, and paint a bright color around the holes. Targets and beanbags are also available through retail outlets.

☐Toss or hand-bat a balloon.

"Hal, who was once a league bowler, is no longer able to participate, but he enjoys watching the action from a table right behind us. We buy him a hamburger, fries and a soda, chat with him frequently, and he has a great time."

Be not disturbed at being misunderstood;
be disturbed rather at not being understanding.
—Chinese Proverb

Gardening

Whether indoors or out in the garden, plants are some of life's greatest miracles. With a little assistance from caregivers, AD family members and patients can experience this miracle in their lives.

☐ Add fertilizer or soil amendments to planting areas — in ground, pots, barrels or planter boxes.

☐ Buy a plant kit — bulb in a box or planter, or others.

☐ Create deck gardens in barrels or wood planter boxes.

☐ Dig weeds.

☐ Raise African violets. **Caregiver**: African violets are easy to grow and propagate indoors, and they are available in many colors.

☐ Grow herbs in barrels or pots on a deck, porch or indoors for use in cooking or sachets.

☐ Hoe.

☐ Make stepping stones from kits.

☐ Mist plants indoors and out.

☐ Paint flower pots. **Caregiver**: Choose favorite colors, use stencils or create freehand designs.

☐ Pick vegetables, berries, and fruit. **Caregiver**: No ladders please!

☐ Place fertilizer sticks in potted plants.

☐ Plant a terrarium.

☐ Plant a rock garden using succulents and drought-tolerant flowers.

☐Plant bulbs in pots for indoor spring blooms.
☐Plant flowers in a window box.
☐Plant seeds . . . in outdoor beds, planter boxes, pots, or egg cartons. Plant vegetables in raised beds or in containers that can be easily moved for ease in sit-down harvesting.
☐Pot plants.
☐Prune/clip/pick dead leaves and flowers.
☐Put fanciful, weather-resistant figurines among the flowers.
☐Put whirlygigs or pinwheels along the garden path.
☐Select seeds from catalogs.
☐Set up a reflection/gazing ball.
☐Shovel and turn soil.

"A 96-year-old friend planted and harvested a beautiful garden with the aid of his walker and help from friends who rototilled the soil and hauled heavy bags of fertilizer."

☐Sprout an avocado seed in a dish of water.
☐Sprout beans in a jar. **Caregiver**: It's fun to watch them grow, and bean sprouts are delicious in salads and oriental dishes.
☐Start new plants from slips.
☐Tie plants to stakes and trellises.
☐Transplant seedlings.
☐Visit a nursery.
☐Water indoor and outdoor plants.
☐Weed flower beds.

Graduations

Graduations represent academic achievement and are occasions to honor graduates and their families, and to reminisce about our own graduations. Encourage your AD family member to think back to his or her graduation, and to praise recent graduates.

☐ Attend a graduation ceremony. **Caregiver**: The usually brief, relaxed graduations for young children (nursery school or kindergarten) can be especially fun.

☐ Attend a baccalaureate service.

☐ Buy a gift or greeting card for a graduate.

☐ Call a graduate and congratulate him or her.

☐ Decorate a purchased graduation card with glitter.

☐ Invite a graduating student to your home for cookies and punch. Ask him or her about future dreams and goals.

☐ Mail a congratulatory card to a graduate.

☐ Pick a bouquet of flowers for a girl graduate.

☐ Talk about your graduation. How old were you when you graduated from high school or college? What year was that? From what town and school did you graduate? What was your graduation like (month, time of day, weather)? Was your graduating class large or small? Did you go to a party after the ceremony? What kind of car were you driving that year? What music was popular?

☐Wrap a gift for a graduate.

> *"Vern recalled proudly that he was the first member of his family to graduate from high school. 'It was a small town and about half the audience was related to me,' he said."*

The Great Depression (1929-1930s)

This major financial tragedy began around the time of the stock market crash in October of 1929 and continued through the 1930s. Families in every state and socio-economic class were affected, and it's likely that your AD family member or patient will remember life experiences during that devastating American struggle.

☐Browse through a family photo album from the 1930s. Who are the people in the pictures? What was their life like? Where did they work? How much were they paid? What did they do to survive?

☐Look through a pictorial book on the Great Depression. Which scenes resemble your experiences? How do the pictures make you feel?

☐Share a story about the Great Depression with a child or classroom of children.

☐Talk about life during the Great Depression. How old were you at that time? Where did your family live? What was the hardest thing about those years? What things did your family do to save money — eat less, wear hand-me-down clothes, grow your own food, work longer days, walk instead of traveling in a motorized vehicle? What jobs were available? What happy things do you remember? How did the Depression change your life then and in years to come?

☐Watch the classic movie *Grapes of Wrath*. Did you ever travel, work, or live like this or know people who did?

Greeting Cards

A greeting card is a friendly message from someone who is absent. Creating, sending and/or receiving greeting cards are rewarding experiences.

☐Add decorative touches to purchased greeting cards using glitter, stickers, or three-dimensional cutouts attached with double-backed tape.

☐Buy a greeting card for a friend.

☐Create simple greeting cards with construction paper, felt-tipped pens, pre-typed verses, stamps, or computer-generated designs.

☐Decorate greeting card envelopes with felt-tipped pens or stamps.

☐ Display a few greeting cards that you have saved from years gone by (birthday cards on your birthday, Valentine's cards on Valentine's Day, etc.)

☐ Make a list of people you want to send cards to.

☐ Put postage stamps on cards to be mailed.

☐ Use a binder, portable file, or decorate a box to save greeting cards. **Caregiver**: It's fun to look at the colorful cards, refreshing memories of friends and family members who sent them.

☐ Write the names of friends or family members on sticky notes and attach them to the cards you plan to send to them.

☐ Talk about your greeting card collection. Which are your favorites? Do you recall greeting cards you received as a child? Did you make cards at school for your mother on Mother's Day or your parents at Christmas? Did you buy or make your Valentine's cards? How much did cards cost when you were young? How much to mail them?

When walking through the forest of life, wise caregivers pause frequently to rest and meditate.

Grocery Shopping

A trip to the grocery store is an excellent adventure for many AD patients. They enjoy being with you and helping with an important household task. While shopping, encourage your AD family member to push the grocery cart. The added support will help him or her feel more secure.

☐At self-serve markets, help unload the grocery cart and bag grocery items.

☐Carry out and help load purchased grocery items in the car.

☐Cut out coupons and pictures of grocery items needed.

☐Help put purchased food in cabinets, refrigerator and freezer and nonfood items in appropriate places.

☐Make a list of groceries to buy.

☐Organize groceries in the cart.

☐Push the grocery cart.

☐Select favorite foods from a list of basic food groups.

☐Select fruit and vegetables.

> *"My friend Charlotte takes my mother-in-law, Hilda, grocery shopping once a week. I look forward to those free hours when I can truly relax and enjoy activities just for me."*

Halloween (October 31)

Halloween, currently one of the most popular celebrations in the United States, originated with the ancient druids in Gaul and Britain, who disguised themselves to hide from evil spirits and gave them treats to appease them. Centuries later, the Catholic Church set aside November 1 as All Saints' Day, or All Hallow's Day, to honor all saints who had no special day of their own. The evening before was called All Hallows' Even, which eventually was shortened to Halloween when the two festivals merged.

☐ Bake and decorate Halloween cookies.

☐ Buy or gather mini-pumpkins, gourds and fall leaves for table decorations.

☐ Carve jack-o-lanterns.

☐ Decorate a room with black and orange streamers or balloons.

☐ Display Halloween decorations on walls, using double-backed tape or reusable adhesive such as Handi-Tak.

☐ Dress in a harvest- or fun Halloween costume.

☐ Fill a bowl with candy, in-the-shell peanuts, or other sugarless treats.

☐ Hand out treats to children Halloween evening.

☐ Make a scarecrow to display in the yard.

☐ Play *Halloween bingo*. ($2.40 for four double-sided playing cards and 124 game pieces, Oriental Trading Co.)

☐ Prepare bags of treats for trick-or-treaters.

☐ Share memories of happy past Halloweens and

traditions observed.

☐Visit an elementary school to watch the children's costume parade. **Caregiver**: Call the school a couple weeks before Halloween to obtain approval to attend and confirm precise location, date and time of costume parade.

☐Visit a pumpkin farm.

☐Wear a Halloween pin on your lapel or collar.

Hanukkah (Date varies)
Festival of Rededication; Festival of Lights

Hanukkah recalls the victory of the Jews over Syrian King Antiochus IV and his armies, a 23-year battle in which the Jews were outnumbered 6 to 1. In 165 B.C. the victorious Jews rededicated Jerusalem's Holy Temple, which had been desecrated by the Syrians. According to Talmudic tradition, at the rededication there was only enough oil for the menorah to burn for one day but, miraculously, it burned for eight days. To commemorate this miracle, an eight-day festival was declared. The joyous celebration begins on the 25th day of the Hebrew month of Kislev, which usually occurs in December. Please note that Hanukkah commemorates the miracle of the oil, not the military victory.

☐Attend a Hanukkah party.

☐Attend religious services.

☐Call someone to wish them a happy Hanukkah.

☐Clean and polish the menorah.

☐Light candles.

☐Make a list of gifts to give to special children.
☐Make a festival of lights centerpiece.
☐Pray traditional Hanukkah prayers.
☐Put candles in the menorah.
☐Send Hanukkah cards to family and friends.
☐Sing Hanukkah songs.
☐Spin a dreidel.
☐Talk about past Hanukkahs. What is your happiest Hanukkah memory? Has the celebration changed since you were a child? What gifts did you receive?
☐Wrap gifts.

History

Many AD patients' long-term memories contain a wealth of fascinating and valuable information about historic events during their lifetimes. Tap into this data base to learn, love and laugh.

☐Chuckle over Burma Shave verses. **Caregiver**: Most seniors recall with pleasure the Burma Shave jingles once placed along roadways, and many can still recite their favorites.

> **No lady . . .**
> **Likes to dance . . .**
> **Or dine . . .**
> **Accompanied by . . .**
> **A porcupine . . .**
> *Burma Shave*

To refresh memories even more, order a book

of all the old Burma Shave jingles, *Verse by the Side of the Road,* from the American Safety Razor Company.

☐Join a historical society. **Caregiver**: Membership benefits often include a newsletter containing stories about local history, interesting presentations, picnics, day trips, and relaxing opportunities to visit with other members.

> *"My neighbor Fannie, who is over 80, has a poor short-term memory, but she still recalls incredible details about the history of the community in which she grew up. She loves going to our historical group's meetings and sharing her stories."*

☐Subscribe to a magazine featuring information and photos related to U.S. history — *American Heritage,* or others.

☐Take a walking tour of historic sites to enjoy fresh air and learn about history. **Caregiver**: Many historical societies give docent-led tours of historic buildings and sites, and some offer brochures for self-guided tours. Watch the newspaper for announcements of upcoming tours or call your local historical society for a calendar of events. Most tours are fund-raisers and, therefore, charge a fee, but some are free or low-cost to the disabled. **Caregiver**: Before taking a tour, it's a good idea to call for details on how vigorous the walk will be — whether there will be steep streets, stairs or other physical challenges. This is especially important if your family member uses a cane, walker or wheelchair.

☐ Talk about historic events that happened during your lifetime. What historic event do you remember most? Was it fun or frightening? How old were you when it happened? Did your family do anything special or unusual because of this event?

Host/Hostess

Mentally challenged family members whose social skills remain active often enjoy helping to arrange and host gatherings.

☐ Arrange bouquets of flowers.

☐ Arrange mini-bouquets (one or two flowers, with or without additional greenery, in tiny vases or bottles) for place settings.

☐ Call a family member or friend and invite him or her to visit you.

☐ Decide where guests should sit at the dinner table.

☐ Dust furniture and, if outdoors, cushions.

☐ Fill small bowls with candy and nuts.

☐ Greet guests as they arrive.

☐ Help make and arrange place cards.

☐ Prepare simple snacks — cheese spread on

crackers, chips and dip, stuffed celery.
☐Seal and mail invitations.
☐Serve cookies, drinks or hors d'oeuvres to
    guests.
☐Share photos and, if appropriate, recent family
    cards and letters.
☐Select a good location outside for visiting.
☐Take guests on a tour of the house or garden.

Housework

*Helping with household tasks and being praised for jobs
well done reassures AD family members that they are
still productive human beings who are contributing
something valuable to those they love.*

☐Arrange small pillows on a sofa.
☐Brush crumbs from kitchen or dining table.
☐Clean the clothes dryer lint screen.
☐Clean stove top.
☐Clean windows and mirrors.
☐Dust furniture. **Caregiver**: Use a dust cloth
    misted with spray wax, or wear soft cotton,
    wax-misted work gloves for this task.
☐Dust mop the floor.
☐Fluff bed pillows.
☐Fold laundry.
☐Hang up clothes.
☐Load dishwasher.
☐Polish brass or silver objects.

☐Shake out throw rugs.
☐Sprinkle carpet freshener on the floors prior to
  vacuuming.
☐Sweep floors.

> *"My mother sweeps the kitchen*
> *over and over again each day."*

☐Sweep the front porch.
☐Sweep spiderwebs from corners using a broom
  or long-handled brush.
☐Vacuum.
☐Wash and dry dishes.
☐Wipe counters.

Independence Day (July 4)

*This United States holiday commemorates the adoption
of the Declaration of Independence on July 4th, 1776.
The day is popularly called Fourth of July. Celebrate by
counting the blessings of bygone Fourths and making
this day memorable.*

☐Go to a parade or watch one on television.
☐Listen to patriotic music — military bands or
  other versions of marches, the *Star Spangled
  Banner*, *My Country Tis of Thee*, *America the
  Beautiful* and other familiar songs.
☐Have a picnic.
☐Put up, take down and fold the flag.

☐Talk about Fourth of Julys during your child-hood. Did you go to a parade? Have a picnic? Shoot off fireworks? What kind of fireworks?

☐Watch fireworks. **Caregiver**: Most AD patients will not be interested in seeing the real thing, but they may enjoy a televised special featuring fireworks and patriotic music.

Japanese New Year
(January 1)

The New Year celebration is the most popular holiday on the Japanese calendar. Traditionally, home entrances are decorated with pine boughs and straw garlands to ward off the entrance of anything impure. Families gather to feast on special soup and sake to ensure good fortune, long life and to cleanse them of unhappy memories remaining from the old year. Many people also visit shrines to pray for good fortune in the coming year.

☐Arrange fresh or silk flowers in a new vase.

☐Call someone and wish him or her a happy new year.

☐Display a collection of origami forms, dolls or other precious items in a place of honor.

☐Help prepare and serve special food and drink.

☐Invite a friend to your home for tea and cookies.

☐Listen to Japanese music.

❑Look through a family photo album. **Caregiver**: Identify and record people, places and dates, and other information.

❑Play *sugoroku* (a Japanese game like parcheesi).

❑Play *fuku warai* with family members. **Caregiver**: This game is similar to pin-the-tail-on-the-donkey. Blindfolded players try to put features in appropriate places on a blank face. *Fuku warai* can be purchased at import shops or online.

❑Prepare pine boughs and straw garlands to hang over the entrance to the front door.

❑Read a book or story about Japan or a famous Japanese person.

❑Share the history of your family with a young relative or friend.

❑Share mementos from the past with your family.

❑Talk about past New Year celebrations. What is your favorite New Year memory? How did your family celebrate when you were a child? What games did you play? What did your kites look like?

❑Teach a young child to spin a top, or watch older children spin tops.

❑Visit a shrine to pray for good fortune in the coming year.

❑Visit friends and wish them a happy new year.

❑Watch children fly kites.

❑Wrap a small gift as a surprise for a special person in your life.

Jewelry

Women have worn and treasured jewelry since ancient times, and many ladies continue to enjoy wearing and sorting through their baubles long after they become mentally frail.

☐ Arrange earrings in a compartmentalized jewelry box or on an earring stand.

☐ Choose favorite jewelry to wear each day or for special occasions.

☐ Have a ring cleaned at a jewelry store. **Caregiver**: Watch for special offers when stores provide this service free of charge.

☐ Polish silver jewelry.

☐ Sort through your jewelry box. **Caregiver**: If your AD family member doesn't have jewelry or needs more to sort, you can buy inexpensive costume pieces at thrift stores, discount stores, and at yard sales. You may find that even children's plastic beads will make your lady happy.

☐ Talk about a favorite piece of jewelry. Why is it your favorite? Where did you get it? On what occasions did you wear it?

☐ Visit a craft fair or mart and watch jewelry being made.

☐ Visit a jewelry store.

> **A moment of joy is a precious jewel set in the golden links of time.**

Martin Luther King, Jr. Day
(January 17)

Civil rights leader Dr. Martin Luther King, Jr. (1929-1968) was committed to justice and moral righteousness. During January, he is remembered with prayers, marches and volunteerism, and young people are challenged to emulate him.

❏Attend community memorial services.

❏Go to the library and read a story or short book about the Rev. Martin Luther King, Jr.

❏Invite teenagers to visit or help you as one of their activities in the Martin Luther King, Jr. National Kindness & Justice Challenge. **Caregiver**: Contact local schools requesting specific services.

❏Participate in the National Kindness & Justice Challenge by complimenting someone, helping a friend with a task, or doing some other good deed.

❏Tell an inspiring story about your life to a child. Who encouraged you when you were young — a family member, teacher, pastor, youth leader? What is the best thing you have accomplished during your lifetime? What hardships did you, your parents or grandparents overcome? Who were famous people you admired? Did you ever meet a famous person who inspired you?

☐Write on paper, or record on audiotape, acts of kindness and justice you have experienced during your lifetime.

Kitchen Tasks

Be sure to give simple, step-by-step directions for all kitchen tasks. It helps to work closely with AD family members and patients, offering encouragement, chatting about happy subjects, or singing familiar songs.

☐Arrange a bouquet of flowers on the table.
☐Arrange canned goods on a shelf.
☐Brush crumbs from the table.
☐Carry vegetable parings to the compost pile.
☐Carry trash to the garbage can.
☐Dust dishes and glassware before a special breakfast, brunch, lunch, dinner or party.
☐Fold kitchen towels and dishcloths.
☐Fold napkins at mealtime.
☐Load the dishwasher.
☐Mop the floor.
☐Organize silverware in a drawer. **Caregiver**: If this is a favorite activity, mix the utensils from time to time so they need organizing again.
☐Organize measuring cups and spoons, placing smaller items in larger ones.
☐Organize the "catchall" drawer — rubber bands, coupons, paper clips, twisty-ties, etc.
☐Put a colorful tablecloth — appropriate for the

season or holiday — on the table.
☐Put labels on canning jars or freezer containers.
☐Rinse dirty dishes.
☐Scoop bagged sugar and flour into canisters.
☐Set the table — place mats, napkins, utensils, plates, glasses.
☐Set out bowls, measuring cups and spoons, and ingredients in preparation for baking and cooking.
☐Sweep the floor.
☐Take dirty dishes from the table to the sink after meals.
☐Wash and dry dishes.
☐Wheel the garbage can to the driveway for pickup.
☐Wipe counters.

Korean War/Korean Conflict (1950-1953)

People over 45 are most likely to remember events during this war between North Korea (aided by Communist China) and South Korea (aided by the U.S. and other United Nations members forming a United Nations armed force).

☐Listen to pop music from the early 1950s. What memories do these songs bring back?
☐Look through an album of photographs taken during the Korean War era. **Caregiver**: Iden-

tify people and places and record them on or beside the appropriate photos.

☐ Talk about your Korean War military service. In which branch of the military did you serve? How old were you? Where did you receive your military training? What was your job? Where were you located? What might have happened if you hadn't done your job correctly? Were you in combat? What things did your family and friends do to encourage and support you while you were overseas — write letters, send gifts, food, clothing and snapshots? Did you receive love letters from a guy or girl back home? Which were your favorite things to receive? How long were you in the military? When were you discharged and what was your rank at that time? How did you feel when the war ended?

☐ Talk about your life as a civilian during the Korean War. How old were you? Were you frightened by the war? What did you and your friends do to help encourage and support servicemen — entertain them, sponsor dances, participate in fund raisers and letter-writing campaigns, make popcorn balls, cookies, and candy to send in Christmas packages, knit mittens and socks, or other activity?

☐ Tape record a story or stories about your life during the Korean War.

Kwanzaa
(December 26-January 1)

This festive, nonreligious holiday has been celebrated in the United States since 1966. During the seven-day celebration, African-Americans reflect upon and honor their ancient African heritage by lighting a candle each night, focusing upon one of seven principles: unity, self-determination, collective work and responsibility, cooperative economics, purpose, creativity and faith. The candles are arranged by colors, which are symbolic — three red candles on the right (for the blood shed in the struggle for freedom), three green candles on the left (for the fertile lands of Africa), and one black candle in the middle (for the color of the people).

☐ Arrange candles in proper color order.
☐ Blow out candles at the end of the evening's celebration.
☐ Buy appropriate colored candles.
☐ Call a family member or friend to wish him or her a happy Kwanzaa.
☐ Fill a bowl with fruits, nuts, and an ear of corn for every child present at your celebration.
☐ Give an educational gift to a child.
☐ Help prepare food for the feast.
☐ Listen while a child reads you a story about African-American history.
☐ Mail a Kwanzaa greeting to someone you love.
☐ Put candles in a Kwansaa candle holder (*kinara*).

☐Read a book or story about a famous African-American.

☐Set the table for the evening feast.

☐Share the story of your African-American heritage with a child.

Labor Day
(First Monday in September)

The first Labor Day parade was sponsored by the Knights of Labor and held on September 5, 1882, in New York City. In 1887 Oregon became the first state to adopt the holiday, which honors working men and women.

While we're on the subject of labor, don't forget the children. In years gone by, before child labor laws were enacted and monitored, children worked at a greater variety of jobs than they do today. You may discover that your family member or patient worked in a home business, on the farm, or in a factory, field or shop.

☐Attend a local parade or watch a special Labor Day program.

☐Clean, repair and sharpen hand tools.

☐Go on a picnic with friends or family members you have worked with.

☐Talk about important work you have done during your lifetime. What work did you do as a child, teen, young adult, adult? What was your most important work? What was your favorite work? How much were you paid for your work? How were you paid — by the hour, day, or week? How did you get to work — on foot, car, bus, street car, train?

❑ Talk about your parents or grandparents work. How was their work different from yours? Did you ever visit your parents or grandparents at their jobs? Did you help them?

❑ Work in the garden or yard.

❑ Visit a hardware store and buy a new tool.

❑ Visit the library and find a book about the type work you did.

> *"We were surprised to learn from Dad that Great Aunt Lily was orphaned as a baby and had to work in a garment factory when she was a young child."*

> *"Mother told us that she helped harvest green beans when she was growing up, and for each full basket, she was paid a silver dollar."*

Still are the ships that in haven ride,
Waiting fair winds or a turn of the tide . . .
Bravely the ships in the tempest tossed,
Buffet the waves till the sea be crossed . . .
Oh, weary hearts, that yearn for sleep,
Look, and learn from the ships of the deep!
—Francis W. Bourdillon

Laundry

As every homemaker knows, there is no end to laundry. A helping hand is always welcome, and the helper enjoys doing something useful.

☐Check clothing for missing buttons.
☐Clean or dust washer and dryer with a damp cloth.
☐Hand-wash lingerie and socks.
☐Fold laundry, perhaps the same basketful over and over again if this is a favorite activity.
☐Hang delicate items on a portable indoor rack.
☐Hang laundry on an outside line to dry.
☐Iron clothes or, even easier, only flat items.
   Caregiver: Avoid this activity if there is any possibility your AD family member may injure himself or herself.
☐Load dirty clothes in a laundry basket in preparation for a trip to the laundromat.
☐Match pairs of socks.
☐Measure and pour detergent in the washer.
☐Put dirty laundry in the washer.
☐Put fabric softener liquid in the washer or a fabric softener sheet in dryer.
☐Put wet wash in the dryer.
☐Put clean laundry in drawers or closets.
☐Separate laundry that needs to be ironed.
☐Set or monitor a minute timer for the period a stain-release product should remain on soiled spots.

☐Sort laundry for washing.
☐Spray or pour a stain-release product on soiled spots.
☐Take clothes from dryer and pile in laundry basket.

Abraham Lincoln's Birthday
(Born February 12, but now officially celebrated on the third Monday in February, Presidents' Day)

Although commemorated for many years, the first officially recognized celebration of Lincoln's birthday was sponsored by the Republican Club of New York and held at a dinner in Delmonico's Restaurant in 1887.

☐Decorate a wall with cutouts of a log cabin, stovepipe hat, Civil War-era scenes, soldiers from the North and South, and/or pictures of Abraham and Mary Lincoln. **Caregiver**: Buy preprinted books or draw your own pictures.
☐Display the American flag.
☐Draw a log cabin, stovepipe hat or Abraham Lincoln.
☐"Build" a log cabin. **Caregiver**: On a pre-printed outline of a log cabin (heavier paper works best), glue or paste brown paper "logs" on the walls, white cotton-ball

"smoke" rising from the chimney, and gray pebble "rocks" in the yard.
□ Talk about Abraham Lincoln. Did you learn about him in school? Was his picture on the wall of your classroom? Did anyone in your family fight in the Civil War? Why was he important?

Magazines

I believe there must be at least one (and in most cases more than one) magazine for every topic in the universe. While that may not be totally accurate, I'm confident you will have no trouble finding just the right magazine to satisfy the interests of your AD family member or patient.

□ Browse through magazines at the grocery store, library or newsstand. Which ones do you like? Why?
□ Buy a favorite magazine or a magazine sub-scription to give as a gift to a friend.
□ Go to a secondhand or thrift shop and look through old magazines. **Caregiver**: Take ad-vantage of bargain prices to reminisce to your heart's content.
□ Make a scrapbook of favorite pictures cut from magazines. **Caregiver**: Narrow subject matter as much as possible — dogs, hats, men work-ing, trucks — but be prepared to make it

broader — animals, clothing, men or people, vehicles — if finding appropriate pictures becomes difficult.

☐ Talk about magazines you recall from years gone by — *Life, Look, The Saturday Evening Post*, or others.

Magnifying Glasses

Magnifying glasses are available in a wide range of styles and prices. For a few dollars you can buy small pocket and hand-held magnifiers. Prices increase for special features and added quality — small- and large-diameter lenses, varying lens powers, unlit or lighted with battery or electricity, table models, headgear attachments, tilt up magnifying lenses to wear over eyeglasses, and others. I recommend starting with something simple and inexpensive.

☐ Collect several objects and examine them through a magnifying glass. **Caregiver**: Use a small basket or box to gather a leaf, flower, tree bark, rock, piece of fabric, string, coin, and other items. Make an adventure of the gathering process, taking time to look around and talk about which things might be interesting to examine under a magnifying lens. If your family member tires easily, make this a two-part process: 1) collect objects and 2) view them later.

☐Examine photos in a pictorial history portraying the eras in which you have lived, then look at them through a magnifying glass. **Caregiver**: Encourage your family member to describe what he sees.

☐Look at old family photos through a magnifying glass. **Caregiver**: This is especially helpful for aging eyes, but younger people will also enjoy details they may otherwise have missed.

☐Share the fun of using a magnifying glass with a child. **Caregiver**: Remind your AD family member that many children have never experienced this pleasant experience of discovery.

Mail

Everyone enjoys receiving mail, and actively maintaining this method of communication may help your AD family member stay more alert and connected to relatives and friends, especially those who live far away.

☐Bring mail from the postal box into the house.

☐Buy stamps at the post office.

☐Carry mail to the postal box, and put the red flag up if it is a rural box.

☐File postcards, greeting cards and letters in a binder. **Caregiver**: Use plastic sheet protectors and plastic photo/postcard pages to make this task and later viewing easier. Add written comments where appropriate.

❒Collect rubber stamps, ink pads, stickers and colored pens to decorate stationery and envelopes.

❒Organize greeting cards in a box with dividers for various special occasions. **Caregiver**: Organizers can be purchased at stationery stores, online or through Current. Or, decorate a cardboard box and add your own dividers.

❒Photocopy cartoons, recipes, pictures, or poems to include with cards and letters.

❒Read mail. **Caregiver**: If letters don't come in regularly, reread old ones. Contact friends and family to write and send cards, even if they live locally. Consider writing faux letters or cards if your loved one becomes agitated because a special person doesn't maintain regular contact. And don't forget e-mail.

❒Select a greeting card to send to a family member or friend. **Caregiver**: Buy one or choose one from those stored at home.

❒Sign and mail a greeting- or postcard to someone. **Caregiver**: A line or two on the postcard card would be a bonus, but it is not necessary. Don't overlook children in your life. Even those nearby will enjoy receiving postcards.

❒Write a note or letter to a family member or friend. **Caregiver**: If your family member has difficulty writing, encourage him to tell you what he would like to say as you write it down. If he cannot think of anything to write, ask leading questions to encourage recollections.

Make suggestions regarding what to write:
We can tell Vera what the weather is like today. Shall we ask her how she's feeling? Does Uncle Jim have children? How about asking him how his children are? What type work does Sally do? Would you like to ask her if she got the promotion? I bet Jake would enjoy hearing about the flowers you planted last week. Please refresh my memory about what they were and their colors. I love the funny story you told me about the waitress at the coffee shop. May I share that with Bessie? I'm sure it will make her laugh.

Read the note or letter back when you have finished, and praise him or her for writing such a wonderful message.

☐ Shop for postcards and greeting cards. **Caregiver**: Each needs only a signature or brief message, a mailing address, and it's ready to mail. Additional meaningful activities include stuffing the greeting card envelope, sealing it and applying the postal stamp.

☐ Shop for tablets and stationery. **Caregiver**: Lined paper is usually helpful, and decorated sheets are fun. Be careful, however, to choose simple stationery designs that will not confuse your AD family member if he or she will be doing the writing.

Maps/Globes

Maps with larger-than-average print and a good-quality magnifying glass are very helpful when searching for locations, roadways and other geographic details. Lay the opened map on a table for easier viewing.

❏Clip a current events article from a newspaper or magazine and find the location of the event on a world globe or map. **Caregiver**: Newer maps and globes, with current boundaries and names of countries, are most helpful.

❏Collect and display small toy globes.

❏Play "Discovery" using a world globe. **Caregiver**: With eyes closed, ask your AD family member or patient to point to a place on a world globe. (Spinning the globe slowly adds to the fun.) Ask, "What did you discover?"

A "correct" answer may be simple. For instance, "This island is in the Pacific Ocean," "This island is in the ocean," or "This is an island." If he or she cannot answer, share a fact or two from your knowledge or research the place in an encyclopedia or online to learn facts.

❏Put together a jigsaw puzzle of the United States. **Caregiver**: There are a variety of paper and wood puzzles available at toy and variety stores. Some puzzles combine several states per puzzle piece.

❏Name a town, state or country you have thought

about visiting and find it on a map or globe.
❑On a map, find towns, states or countries you've lived in.
❑Using a map, find towns or states lived in by ancestors. **Caregiver**: This is another excellent opportunity to gather family stories.

> "Where in the world shall we go, my friend?
> Around the globe and back again. "

May Day (May 1)

This festival is believed to have its roots in an ancient Roman festival honoring Flora, the goddess of flowers. In European countries and in the United States, May Day was (and still is, in some places) celebrated by dancing around the Maypole, playing games, and delivering surprise baskets of flowers to friends.

❑Arrange flowers in a vase or other container to create a May Day centerpiece.
❑Give flowers to a friend.
❑Make a Maypole collage. **Caregiver**: Help your AD family member cut out and glue a brown or silver "pole" in the middle of a light blue sheet of construction paper. Glue or staple six or more colorful ribbons to the top of the pole and adorn with small silk flowers or flowers cut from magazines.

◻Make a simple bouquet wall decoration. **Caregiver**: Help your family member glue a variety of silk flowers and leaves on a piece of felt. Attach to a dowel, place in a frame, or hang on a wall with tape or Handi-Tak.
◻Pick a bouquet of wild flowers.

> *"Eighty-one-year-old Sarah recalls the happy May Day celebrations of her youth: 'One year I was crowned queen of the maypole. My mother made me a new dress, wove flowers in my braids, and clapped her hands as I danced around the maypole with my friends.'"*

Medical

Many AD patients recall accurate details about the history of their medical care beginning with stories about their birth. Even after their minds begin to falter, they often enjoy talking about their health history, and a medical appointment may be a highlight of life.

◻Attend appropriate free health and medical presentations.
◻Collect magazines around your home and donate them to your doctor's office waiting room or to a hospital.
◻Eat breakfast, lunch or dinner in a hospital cafeteria. **Caregiver**: Meals are generally inexpensive, and some medical facilities offer

even lower rates and special meals for seniors.

☐Listen to your heart through a stethoscope.

☐Look at relatives' photographs in a family album and tell what illnesses or health problems they had. **Caregiver**: Document this information for your family's medical history. It will be interesting information and, more important, might prove invaluable to you and future generations.

☐Mail a picture post card to your doctor. He or she will probably display it on a wall or in an album. Look for it on your next office visit.

☐Pose for a snapshot with your doctor, dentist, ophthalmologist, physical therapist, chiropractor, or other healthcare provider. **Caregiver**: As a helpful reminder for your AD family member, label a copy of the photo and frame it, or place it in a convenient album. Give or mail photo copies to friends or relatives who are interested in your AD family member's health and his or her healthcare providers.

"My father remembers the doctor who has cared for him for over twenty years, but he doesn't recall his dentist of three years from one visit to the next."

☐Take a small gift to your doctor or office staff — a book, juicy apple, fresh vegetables or fruit from your garden, potted plant, thank-you card, box of candy.

☐Talk about your past medical care. What was medical care like when you were a child? Do you remember the name of your family doctor back then? Did he or she make house calls? Were you born in a hospital or at home? Were you or any member of your family ever hospitalized? Did you ever have an operation? What medicines did you take when you were a youngster? What were they for? What folk remedies were used in your home?

> *"Julio, one of 10 children, says his mother tied strings of garlic around his and his siblings' necks to ward off colds."*

> *"Ninety-year-old Angus recalls that his mother dosed him with bitter home-brewed tonic every spring, and when he had pink eye, his father wiped fresh urine on his eyes as a curative. It worked, Angus assures me."*

"The irony of it. My mother, a woman who based her entire life on control, has now lost all of it, mind and body. Once proud and unapproachable, she has returned to her childhood. In letting go, she has found love. . . . For me, it has been two years of crises. Rent the house, pay the bills, deal with doctors . . . hire the extra caregivers . . . change doctors, retrain caregivers, hire a new daily companion . . . But most of all, hold my mom. Hold on for dear life."
—Susan Pringle-Cohan, The Gift from Cartwheels on the Faultline

---

Memorial Day
(Last Monday in May, formerly May 30)

This holiday originated in 1868 when Gen. John A. Logan, Commander in Chief of the Grand Army of the Republic (GAR), set aside "Decoration Day" for decorating the graves of Union soldiers. The name was eventually changed to "Memorial Day" and now honors the dead of all wars. Some southern states observe Memorial Day on different dates — April 26, May 10, and June 3.

☐ Call someone who served in the military and thank him or her.

☐ Display wartime mementos — awards and medals, military uniforms, ration tickets, family letters, figurines, service flags, souvenir plates, mugs, pillows, pins.

☐ Look at or display family photos of men and women who served in the military.

☐ Pick a bouquet of flowers and arrange in a vase.

☐ Put up, take down and fold the flag.

☐ Talk about memorable military service, brave deeds done, and honors received.

☐ Visit the cemetery and put flowers on the graves of deceased loved ones who served in the military. **Caregiver**: Some families clean up and decorate the graves of all relatives on this day.

☐ Watch a parade in person or on television.

☐ Wear red, white and blue.

Memory Boxes

Memory boxes are nothing new, but I discovered their usefulness for AD patients at the facility where my father participates in Day Club activities and spends occasional overnights as part of the respite care program. Dad loves his memory box, which contains his name and former occupation in bold print, and a few mementos from his past. When he stays overnight, the memory box is hung on the wall outside his room. Dad has trouble remembering and locating the room number on the door, but he recognizes his memory box. He is very proud of it and never tires of talking about the objects in it and how they relate to his life. I enjoy other residents' memory boxes, too, which poignantly remind me of each individual's unique qualities and value.

A portable memory box can be moved so the AD patient may sit and leisurely browse through memorabilia and photographs.

Whether stationary or portable, a memory box is also an excellent home resource. It serves the above purposes and significantly honors your AD family member and his or her contributions to society.

"Only those who have cared for an Alzheimer's patient understand how difficult the job is. In my opinion, all AD caregivers are saints, and those who care for family members at home are super-saints."
—H.H., social worker

Portable Memory Box

A portable memory box can be as simple as a small, sturdy cardboard carton or plastic box containing a few memorable objects. On the other hand, you might prefer or need something larger, especially if memorabilia include big or irregularly shaped objects such as ice skates, model airplanes, quilt blocks, sewing baskets, school yearbooks, stamp collections, tools or trophies.

Stationary Memory Box

A stationary memory box remains permanently or semipermanently in the same place — on a wall, shelf, or other area where it can be viewed easily. When hanging it on a wall, place it at a comfortable eye level for your family member, better lower than higher because many AD patients have difficulty looking up. In addition, make sure lighting around and on the memory box is adequate.

Shadow box frames with glass fronts are available in a variety of sizes and prices at craft shops, professional picture framers, and other stores. Gather several favorite

> "Home is a concept in [Mother's] mind. Going home to her is a journey in time, not space . . . She is completely in the present, the past a tangled thicket of dreams and the future incomprehensible." —Susan Pringle Cohan, The Gift from Cartwheels on the Faultline

items in contrasting colors, sizes and shapes, and experiment until you find a combination that is esthetically pleasing.

The list of potential items for your memory box is endless: autographed baseballs, books, coins, desk name plates, doilies, dolls, fabric, figurines, game pieces, gloves, greeting cards, jewelry, kitchen utensils, letters, professional business cards and name tags, military insignia, passports, photographs of family, pets and on-the-job scenes, picture postcards, playing cards, prayer books, silk flowers, sports memorabilia, stitchery, teacups, tools . . .

A glass-topped display table for memorabilia can also serve as a memory box. With a recessed space below the glass hinged-lid, these tables are available at furniture stores in small to substantial sizes. If your AD family member doesn't care to handle objects frequently, the display table may meet his or her needs.

❐Decorate your portable memory box with wrapping paper, stamps, stickers, cutouts, paint, or glitter.

❐Help select and place items in your memory box.

❐Invite a family member or friend to look at items in your memory box. **Caregiver**: Encourage visitors to bring small gifts that can be added to the memory box.

❐Put your name on or in your memory box. **Caregiver**: Your family member may write his name in bright ink on a label or directly on

the portable memory box, or paste on a preprinted or computer designed label. For the clear plastic, stationary memory box, place a fairly large, easy-to-read name card inside.
☐ Talk about the items in your memory box. Which is your favorite item?

Military Service

Serving in the military is a memorable experience for most servicemen and -women, and many AD patients enjoy activities that call back memories of those youthful, life-changing years. In addition to the ideas below, see suggestions under specific military actions (e.g., WWII, Korean War) in which your family member or patient may have been involved.

☐ Attend a Veterans of Foreign Wars (VFW) reunion.
☐ Attend local VFW meetings and programs. **Caregiver**: Activities may include lectures, readings and slide shows by veterans, Boy/Girl Scouts, or others; drill team presentations; recognition days for POWs/MIAs; shuffleboard or horseshoe pitching tournaments; picnics and potlucks.
☐ Demonstrate your military salute. With whom did you exchange salutes?
☐ Look at photographs taken during your military service. **Caregiver**: Identify and document

people, places, dates, and relevant comments.

☐Read the local VFW post newsletter.

☐Send a greeting card to a serviceperson through the Dear Abby program.

☐Subscribe to the VFW Magazine.

☐Talk about your military basic training. Was basic training easy or difficult? What did you like least? What time did you get up in the morning? How were you trained and what were you trained to do? What was the military method of making your bed? What was the most important thing you learned?

☐Talk about your military experience. In which branch of the armed services did you serve? When? Where? How old were you? How did your family feel about your entering military service? What did you like best about being in the military? What did you like least?

☐Talk about your military uniforms. How many uniforms, hats, shoes, socks, etc. were issued to you? What colors were they and what did they look like? Were they comfortable? What were some of the military rules about when to wear different uniforms and how they should look? How did you keep your uniforms clean and pressed? How often did you polish and shine your shoes? What happened if your uniform wasn't spick-and-span during inspection?

☐Talk about your superior officers. Who was

your favorite? Why? Who was your least favorite? Why?

☐Talk about your military buddies. Who was your best friend? Where did you meet? What things did you do together? What was the wildest or most daring thing you did with your buddies?

☐Visit with an old buddy or new military friend.

> "There is something magnificent in having a country to love. It is almost like what one feels for a woman. Not so tender, perhaps, but to the full as self-forgetful."
> —James Russell Lowell, 1865

Miscellaneous Fun

Some successful activities spring from surprising resources. Let your imagination take wing to come up with more.

☐Black out prices or bar codes on household products with a marking pen, or place decorative stickers over them. Why? They look so much neater that way.

☐Bundle twigs for the fireplace. Tie the twig bundles with twine or place in paper bags for fire starters. **Caregiver**: As you would with children, keep matches safely hidden.

☐Crack and shell walnuts or other nuts. Put some in small containers to give to friends and relatives, or freeze nuts for later use.

☐ Experience an Alzheimer's Activity Apron. **Caregiver**: The apron is covered with things to touch and manipulate — buttons, zippers, pockets, Velcro fasteners, ribbons to braid. Around $25. Available through Elder Press and NOVITEM Enterprises.

☐ Gather rubber bands from a catchall drawer and put them in plastic baggies.

☐ Mend torn paper products with adhesive tape. If you don't have anything to repair, tear something! Use sheets of plain or printed paper, letters, envelopes, greeting cards, grocery ads, coupons, gift-wrapping, or calendars.

☐ Polish shoes — yours or family members'.

☐ Roll string, twine or yarn into a ball.

☐ Sharpen knives and scissors using a whet stone. **Caregiver**: This activity, which appeals to many men, should be introduced only if your AD family member can safely handle sharp implements.

☐ Stamp borders or your name and address on 8½" x 11" sheets of paper. **Caregiver**: This is busy work, so the sheets need only be free of print on one side. Recycle discardable mail and advertising letters, or ask a local business to give you paper they would otherwise discard.

☐ Put the current date or year on canned goods

and on other pantry products. Write with a marking pen directly on containers or use adhesive labels.

Money

Money makes the world go round, and for many AD patients, the desire to maintain control of their cash remains strong even after the disease steals their logic and calculating abilities. Simple activities involving money, which has been an important part of life since childhood, are often reassuring.

☐Buy a plastic coin counter in which the various denominations (pennies, nickels, dimes, quarters, half-dollars. etc.) roll into appropriate slots.

☐Count coins.

☐Count bills in his wallet or her purse.

☐Go shopping for a piggy bank and save loose change for a special occasion.

☐Make a cash deposit at the bank.

☐Play a simplified *Monopoly* game using play money to buy and sell real estate.

☐Roll coins in bank holders.

☐Place collectible coins (e.g., new state quarters or others) in their special folder slots. Talk about why each coin is special. Which are favorites?

☐Stack coins by denominations — pennies,

nickels, dimes, quarters, etc.

"Dad had lost his ability to tell one coin or bill from another, so when he insisted that he needed 'hundreds of dollars' in his wallet, we filled it with play money and he was satisfied."

"Mother believes people are stealing from her purse so she regularly hides her money. Last night at bedtime we found her cash in a surprising place — stuffed into her Depends."

**"Nothing but Money,
Is sweeter than Honey."**
—Benjamin Franklin, 1735

Mother's Day
(Second Sunday in May)

Mother's Day was originated by Miss Anna M. Jarvis of Philadelphia, and the holiday was first observed on May 10, 1908 in Philadelphia, Pennsylvania, and Grafton, West Virginia. Six years later, President Woodrow Wilson proclaimed the second Sunday in May for public observance of Mother's Day. Today, children of all ages honor their mothers with cards and gifts on this day.

❒Attend religious services. **Caregiver**: Most congregations have special programs and some give small corsages or gifts on this day to honor mothers.

❒Call a young mother and wish her a happy day.

❒Describe your childbearing experiences. **Caregiver**: Women often remember this vividly.

❒Display a photograph of your mother.

❒Make mini-floral arrangements to give to mothers in your family or to friends. **Caregiver**: Have your AD family member pick one or two rosebuds or daisies, add a green leaf or fern, and wrap the arrangement in a damp paper towel and aluminum foil.

❒Play the game "Whose Mother Is This?" **Caregiver**: Take turns naming a mother animal, and her baby — **mare**/foal or colt; **cow**/calf; **deer or doe**/fawn; **sheep or ewe**/lamb; **goose**/gosling, etc.

❒Share happy stories about your mother or children.

❒Share memories of past happy Mother's Days. What traditional activities did you or your mother enjoy on Mother's Day?

❒Wear a corsage to honor your mother or because you are a mother.

"In Angelica's mind, all Mother's Day bouquets are composed of wild sweet peas, a flower her sons always picked for her on that day."

Movie/Television Stars

Actors and the movies and television shows in which they star have a profound impact on people of all ages. Favorites are likely to be remembered and can be utilized for discussion and activities.

☐Help make a list of favorite movie and television stars. What shows were they in? What happy memories do you have about them? How did they dress and wear their hair? Were they funny or dramatic actors?

☐Borrow and read a library book on the history of movies or the story of a movie you enjoyed.

☐Read a book or story about a favorite star.

☐Rent videos or DVDs featuring favorite stars. **Caregiver**: You may find appropriate films through your local library.

☐Share a story about getting a star's autograph, meeting a star, or a star you would like to meet.

☐Talk about your childhood memories of stardom. When you were a child, who was your favorite star? Did you dream of being an actor or actress? Were you ever in a play or movie, or on a television show? What was it like? Did you take dancing, singing or acting lessons?

"Grandpa tells of seeing his first movie around 1914. His uncle bought a projector and folks paid a nickel to sit on a wood bench in the barn and watch the film

projected onto a white sheet hung from the rafters."

"When Lucille was a teenager, she and a group of other female fans mobbed Frank Sinatra. Lucy came away with a piece of the star's necktie."

Movies/Slides

An evening out at the movies is a special event for most of us, but watching home movies or slides can be equally enjoyable. Home productions offer a special advantage for those with impaired hearing: they don't have to worry about missing dialogue or narration. (See "Videos" for additional suggestions on commercially made movies.)

❒Attend community travelogues. **Caregiver**: These movie or slide presentations of national and international trips are usually shown in community theatres or civic organization meeting halls, and tickets are generally inexpensive. Local or regional speakers sometimes provide narration for the presentations and refreshments may be served.

❒Go to a theatre to see an upbeat or humorous movie. **Caregiver**: Select subject matter — a musical, an animal story, or an animated adventure — that would be of interest to your family member. For a truly luxurious experience, go to one of the new theatres with stadium seating and top quality surround sound.

☐Watch old home movies to refresh memories of family members and events. **Caregiver**: Consider putting your home movies on videotape for easier viewing.

Talk about those happy days and people: Grandma, you and Grandpa were the best dancers at my wedding. Where did you learn to waltz like that? When Uncle John began playing T-ball, did you have any idea he would become a major league player? Dad, how many miles did you put on that old truck driving on hunting trips? I loved racing that bicycle with Mike. Did you ride bikes with your brothers and sisters when you were a kid?

☐Have a slide show of past family activities. **Caregiver**: Invite a few close relatives or friends to join you and serve chips and dip and iced tea. Most of us have more slides than home movie footage so plan on at least an hour for relaxed viewing and comments. (If you have thousands of slides as we do, limit the viewing to only a few of them.) Consider putting your slides on videotape or digitizing them onto CD-ROMs for easier viewing.

Talk about past activities during the slide show: That was a beautiful birthday cake you made for my sixth birthday, Mother. Thank you. Dad, what was the largest fish you ever caught? Mom, how did you manage cooking and laundry for all of us on those family camping trips? How many hours did it take you to cut that pile of firewood?

Music

"Of all earthly music, that which reaches the farthest into heaven is the beating of a loving heart."
—Henry Ward Beecher

☐Dance. **Caregiver**: Even walkers and wheelchairs won't stop you from holding hands and moving to the beat and rhythm of the music.

☐Listen to favorite music — radio, records, tapes, CDs. **Caregiver**: Have a portable CD/tape player ("boom box") handy so your loved one can have music wherever he or she wishes.

☐Make up rhyming words to familiar tunes.

☐Play a musical instrument.

☐Play the game "Finish the Song." **Caregiver**: You sing the first line or two of a familiar song, and let your AD family member sing the next line, or as much as he or she wishes to sing. If words are forgotten along the way, make some up or hum the tune. Try a duet.

☐Sing favorite old songs together. **Caregiver**: It doesn't matter if you don't have perfect pitch.

Beautiful music is in the ear of the hearer.

"My eighty-year-old uncle, Frank, brags about his new 'boom box', a term he recently learned from a teenager."

National Alzheimer's Disease Month (November)

"During seasons when my heart is unable to celebrate, my soul clings to the strength and wisdom of others, to ease my pain and give me hope."

—Beatrice Gage

❒Participate in special Alzheimer's-related community activities. **Caregiver**: Contact the national or local Alzheimer's Association for their calendar of events and information.

"When I am with my father, I focus on the present. I remind myself to accept him as he is, not as he was or could be. . . . His world is slowly shrinking, and he is left only with the little things, his memories of mere incidents from years gone by."
—Brenda Avadian, M.A.
Where's My Shoes?
My Father's Walk Through Alzheimer's

Newspapers/Magazines

Like most people, your AD family member is likely to enjoy current publications as well as those that were popular when he or she was young. Relax during these quiet moments together when you are able to discuss current events and reminisce about bygone days.

☐ Clip coupons. File them in an envelope for later use.

☐ Play appropriate games or work puzzles in the children's section. **Caregiver**: It helps to enlarge items on a photocopier.

☐ Read classic old magazines. **Caregiver**: Search for them in libraries, secondhand, antique, and thrift stores. Favorites often include old movie magazines, comic books, *Farmer's Almanac, Field and Stream, Harpers, Ladies' Home Journal, Look, National Geographic, Popular Mechanics, Redbook, Saturday Evening Post, Smithsonian.* Also look for publications of regional interest at the library.

☐ Stack and tie magazines and newspapers for recycling.

☐ Subscribe to newspapers or magazines of special interest. It's fun to receive them in the mail.

☐ Tear off or mark through address labels on magazines that are to be donated.

☐ Visit the library and look through one of the numerous current newspapers or magazines available.

New Year's Day (January 1)

Celebrate the new year with gratitude for blessings, acceptance of challenges, and faith for a brighter future. Resolve to take care of your own needs as well as those of your AD family member, then do it!

❑Bake and decorate a cake with multicolored sprinkles. Place a #1-shaped candle (for the first day of the year) on top.

❑Blow bubbles using bottled bubble fluid. **Caregiver**: To be really fancy, buy bubble fluid in champagne-flute-shaped containers.

❑Cut out pictures from old calendar pages. Donate them to a school, church or organization.

❑Drink sparkling cider out of champagne flutes or other fancy glasses.

❑Watch a football bowl game on television.

❑Watch a New Year's Day parade on television.

❑Wear a New Year's hat and celebrate with a horn or other noisemaker.

"Life is the process of creating special memories with people. These are life's real treasures when we have nothing more."
—Brenda Avadian, M.A.
Where's My Shoes?
My Father's Walk Through Alzheimer's

Office Work

Caregivers who have home-based businesses appreciate help in the office, and AD family members enjoy contributing to important work.

☐ Clean telephones and computer screens.
☐ Clean computer keyboards with a cotton swab and nontoxic cleaning agent.
☐ Dust computers and furniture.
☐ Collate papers.
☐ Fill staplers and paper clip holders.
☐ Fold letters or newsletters.
☐ Organize kitchen supplies.
☐ Photocopy letters and reports.
☐ Punch holes.
☐ Sharpen pencils.
☐ Shred documents.
☐ Stack magazines or catalogs.
☐ Staple sheets of paper.
☐ Stamp envelopes.
☐ Stuff envelopes.
☐ Tear perforated edges from computer paper.
☐ Wash and dry coffee cups.

> "[My mother] doesn't have a clue about where she is, but she can still correct my grammar."
> —Susan Pringle-Cohan, The Gift from Cartwheels on the Faultline

Outdoor Adventures

You don't have to go far to enjoy fresh air and a change of scenery with your AD family member. Both of you will benefit.

☐ Collect shells and driftwood at the seashore.

☐ Enjoy a picnic in the park. **Caregiver**: Take favorite, easy-to-transport snack foods and drinks. If your family member is confined to a wheelchair, take along a folding chair so you can sit together and enjoy the sunshine. Don't forget sunblock and an umbrella or other protection from the sun.

☐ Go to a park to watch children play. **Caregiver**: Encourage your family member to talk about his or her childhood. What type toys did you play on in the park? What was your favorite thing to do at the park?

☐ Relax in a rocking chair on the porch or patio.

☐ Sit in the yard under a shady tree and visit. **Caregiver**: Take a book to read or stitchery to occupy your time if your loved one dozes.

☐ Sun at the beach or by the pool.

☐ Take a ride in the country. **Caregiver**: Driving to new locales can be very relaxing.

☐ Walk. **Caregiver**: A regular (daily, if possible) routine route is usually more reassuring. Pause and point out special beauty — a colorful tree, a fragrant rose, children playing in a sprinkler, men and machinery at work.

"Alice was inclined to focus straight ahead or walk with her head down, but we discovered that if we encouraged her to look at specific things and enthusiastically talked about them, she responded positively."

Passover (Date varies)
Begins at the end of the 14th day of the Jewish month Nisan, usually in March or April

Passover is a joyous, eight-day religious celebration of the Jews' deliverance from bondage in Egypt 3,000 years ago. The Seder, a special feast, is held on the first and second nights of the holy days. During the feast, guests take turns reading the Haggadah, or Passover story.

A ceremonial Seder plate contains symbolic elements: 1) a shank bone of lamb represents the springtime sacrifice of lambs in the Temple in Jerusalem during first harvest; 2) an egg symbolizes life's renewal in the spring; 3) bitter herbs are for the bitterness of slavery in Egypt; 4) charoset represents the mortar that Jews had to mix when building Egyptian pyramids; and 5) parsley dipped in saltwater symbolizes the salty tears of bondage and also the green shoots of hope. Matza, unleavened bread, and wine are also served.

❏Attend synagogue services.
❏Attend Seder.

❏Describe the significance of one or more of the symbolic foods — shank bone of a lamb, an egg, bitter herbs, *charoset* (chopped apples, nuts, and wine), and parsley on the Seder plate.

❏Help prepare the Seder meal.

❏Say a Passover prayer.

❏Sing Passover songs of thanksgiving.

❏Take a turn reading the *Haggadah*.

❏Talk about bygone Passovers. What is your favorite Passover memory? Has the celebration changed since you were a child?

❏Tell the Passover story to a child.

Pearl Harbor Day (Dec. 7)

On December 7, 1941, Japan unexpectedly attacked the U.S. naval base at Pearl Harbor, Oahu, Hawaii. The bombing crippled the Pacific Fleet, killing 2,403 servicemen, destroying 188 airplanes, and damaging or destroying 19 ships. The following day Congress declared war on Japan, launching the U.S. into World War II. The event had a life-changing impact on most Americans.

❏Attend a Pearl Harbor Day memorial service.

❏Name, if you can, one or more of the ships that were damaged or destroyed at Pearl Harbor?

Caregiver: If your family member needs help recalling ship names, mention several and see if they bring back recollections. However, if memories of Pearl Harbor are distressing, avoid this activity.

❏Look at a book about Pearl Harbor.

❏Talk about life experiences during and following the attack on Pearl Harbor. How old were you? Were you, a family member, or friend in Pearl Harbor during the attack? How did life change in America after the Pearl Harbor attack?

❏Wear a flag pin on your collar or lapel in honor of servicemen who were injured or died at Pearl Harbor.

Most Remembered Ships Damaged or Destroyed at Pearl Harbor, December 7, 1941

Arizona	California
Cassin	Downes
Maryland	Oglala
Oklahoma	Pennsylvania
Shaw	Tennessee
Utah	

"For several weeks after the attack on Pearl Harbor, my uncle Gilbert, then 12 years old, and his friends sat on a California hillside each day, fearfully watching for Japanese bombers."

"Love endures long and is patient. . . . "
—1 Corinthians 13:14

Personal Hygiene/Grooming

Men and women with Alzheimer's disease often have difficulty remembering to attend to basic cleanliness, or they have no desire to do so. Don't despair if you face this challenge. With patience, fortitude, and creativity, you may be able to overcome your AD family member's fear, negativity and defiance.

❑Brush teeth.
❑Clean dentures.
❑Clean eyeglasses.
❑Comb or brush hair.
❑File nails.
❑Hand-wash lingerie or socks.
❑Have a manicure or pedicure.
❑Organize toiletries in a colorful box or on a tray.
❑Polish or shine shoes.
❑Polish nails.
❑Put pretty clips or flowers in your hair.
❑Put on or freshen makeup.
❑Select clothing (even one item) to wear.
❑Shave.
❑Splash or spray on after-shave or perfume.

> *"When I suggested that Mother splash on a little cologne, she removed the stopper and shook the bottle with wild abandon, splashing cologne all over herself and me."*

❑Soften hands and face with lotion.

☐Use a lint brush to remove lint from clothing.
☐Visit a beauty salon or barber for a haircut or perm.
☐Wash as much of yourself as possible.
☐Wash combs and brushes.

> *"We hung Dad's collection of caps on his bedroom wall. Each morning after we dress him, he chooses a cap to wear and says, 'How does that look?'"*

> *"When Grandpa first came to live with us, he smelled horrible. He hadn't changed his clothes or bathed for weeks, and when asked if he wanted to clean up, he got angry and said he didn't need to. The problem was finally solved, at least partially, when Grandpa's doctor 'ordered' regular bathtimes."*

Pets/Companion Animals

In politically correct terms, pets are now referred to as "companion animals" and pet owners as "guardians," but I have chosen to use the term "pet" in this edition for readers' convenience. Whatever they are called, these loyal and lovely creatures bring joy into our lives.

☐Bathe the dog.
☐Brush the dog.

☐Change bedding in pet beds.
☐Change the paper in the bird cage.
☐Clean pet hair off furniture.
☐Clean the mat under pet dishes.
☐Cuddle pets.
☐Feed and water pets.
☐Fold pet blankets.
☐Give each pet a snack treat, perhaps at bedtime.
☐Pick up pet toys at the end of the day.
☐Play with pets.
☐Scoop dry dog food from large bags into
    smaller, easier-to-handle containers.
☐Teach pets tricks.
☐Walk the dog.

"When my sister and I began caring for our mother, we thought her dog would be a nuisance, but Tippy turned out to be an angel in disguise. He has a calming effect on Mother that helps us through many difficult moments."

Where Has My Little Dog Gone?
Oh, where, oh, where has my little dog gone?
Oh, where, oh, where can he be?
With his tail cut short and his ears cut long,
Oh, where, oh, where can he be?
—German folk song

Photographs and Albums

Hopefully, you are lucky enough to have family photo albums. If not, or even if you do, consider creating new ones. Choose from among the many delightful album materials currently available in craft stores, and enjoy a relaxing project that will become a family heirloom.

☐ Create a current family photo album. **Caregiver**: Boldly print names and dates below each photo to help refresh memories.

☐ Decorate an acid-free photo box, or buy one, to collect photos.

☐ Look through old family photograph albums. **Caregiver**: Identify and document names, places and dates.

☐ Talk about photos in old albums. Who are the people? What are the events? What exciting things did you do when you were young?

☐ Take pictures of family activities, places you visit (even doctors' office visits), and enjoyable events. **Caregiver**: Put the pictures in an album and write identifying names and dates below each photo. They'll be wonderful memory boosters and subjects for conversation.

> Take a picture, take another,
> Mother, sister, baby brother,
> Someday when you're old and gray,
> They'll remind you of this day.

Politics

Mentally challenged men and women may be as enthusiastic about political candidates and issues as those with sound minds. Savvy caregivers encourage and participate in the political fun.

☐ Attend a town hall meeting where local candidates speak.

☐ Cut out newspaper photos of candidates, glue them on sheets of paper and label them.

☐ Discuss current political issues. **Caregiver**: Select topics that are easily understood and will not be upsetting.

☐ Discuss past political campaigns, specific candidates and issues. Who was the first United States President you voted for? How did people vote back then? Did any family members participate in politics? Which political party do you prefer, and why?

☐ Display a political banner in your home or post a political sign on your lawn.

☐ Drape red, white and blue bunting on your front porch.

☐ Read voter pamphlets.

☐ Seal and stamp envelopes for a local candidate.

☐ Vote. **Caregiver**: If your family member is not competent to vote, he may enjoy your helping him review and check off boxes on the sample ballot.

☐ Watch a political debate on television.

☐ Watch election returns on television.
☐ Wear a pin on your collar promoting your favorite candidate.

"Ninety-eight-year-old Claude enjoyed telling about the day his aunt Bessie learned that Theodore Roosevelt had been elected U.S. President. Swinging her apron, she danced around and shouted, 'Teddy did it! Teddy did it!'"

Postcards

Everyone enjoys picture postcards. Once upon a time they were called "penny postcards" because that is what they cost. Today postcards are more expensive, but they're still a bargain to buy and mail. They are, of course, also fun to receive. How about designing your own postcards? It's easy. Start with booklets of plain postcards available at craft stores.

☐ Buy a pretty postcard to mail to a friend or relative.
☐ Collect postcards in an album or scrapbook.
☐ Color a fuzzy postcard. **Caregiver**: Fuzzy postcards are a bit more expensive but the preprinted patterns, including seasonal themes, are easy to complete and look great when filled in with colored pens.
☐ Decorate a plain postcard with colorful stamps, felt-tipped pens, or colored pencils.

☐Make a list of people you would like to send postcards to.

☐Stencil a design on a postcard and fill in colors. **Caregiver**: If your family member is unable to coordinate stenciling, complete this part of the project and let him or her fill in the design with color. (I recommend colored pencils if smearing is a problem.) Have her sign or initial the finished design (as artists do!).

☐Write a note on a postcard and mail it to a friend or relative. **Caregiver**: You may need to help your AD family member if writing or wording is difficult.

"Shortly after mailing several hand-decorated postcards, we got a call from a distant cousin, thanking Dad for his beautiful card."

"My son Skip travels all over the world on business, and from every location he mails a colorful postcard with a note to his grandmother, which makes her very happy. Using our globe, we show Gran where Skip is and talk about that part of the world."

*"I contacted relatives in various states and asked them to mail postcards of their area to my aunt. She grew teary every time a postcard arrived, saying, 'They **do** remember me.'"*

Presidents of the U.S.

Most of us have vivid memories of U.S. presidents who served during our lifetime and, often, such recollections linger a long time in the impaired mind. Many Americans also know a great deal about our nation's earliest presidents. Use the presidential timelines on pages 136 and 137 to give encouraging hints, refresh old memories, and verify facts.

❑Buy a postcard with a U.S. president or presidential landmark on it and send it to a child.

❑Collect pictures of U.S. presidents, their families, homes, and pets in a scrapbook or album. Label the pictures.

❑Give a coin (5, 10, or 25 cents) for every U.S. president a youngster can name beginning with George Washington. **Caregiver**: Obtain a quantity of coins to keep on hand, and have a list of presidents handy to check the accuracy of the child's recitation.

❑Look through a book about Mount Rushmore. In what state is it located? (South Dakota) Have you visited Mount Rushmore? What do you recall about the United States presidents commemorated there — George Washington, Abraham Lincoln, Thomas Jefferson, Theodore Roosevelt.

❑Name the U.S. presidents you recall, from George Washington to the present.

❑Play a game featuring U.S. presidents. **Care-**

giver: A variety of games are available at stores and online. Encourage children and teens to play games with your AD family member, helping him or her when needed.
☐ Read or listen to a story about a U.S. president.
☐ Sort through coins, separating those with a president's image imprinted on them. How many presidents did you find?
☐ Talk about U.S. presidents. Who was your favorite president? What political party was he a member of? Why did you like him? How old were you when he was president? Did you ever meet or see a U.S. president in person? Do you think the United States will ever have a woman president? Would you like to be president of the United States?
☐ Tell a story to a child about a president, perhaps a story you heard when you were a child — George Washington chopping down the cherry tree or crossing the frozen Potomac during the Revolutionary War; Abraham Lincoln walking miles to return penny change; President Hoover's Hoovervilles, or others.
☐ Visit a presidential monument in Washington, D.C. or other state, or a monument in your community. **Caregiver**: Take a snapshot of the occasion for your photo album.
☐ Watch a video biography of a president.
☐ Watch a video chronicling the presidential carvings on Mount Rushmore.

U.S. Presidents 1789-1901
(1st through 25th)

No.	Term of Office	President	Life Span
01	1789-1797	George **Washington** (Fed)[1]	1732-1799
02	1797-1801	John **Adams** (Fed)	1735-1826
03	1801-1809	Thomas **Jefferson** (R)	1743-1826
04	1809-1817	James **Madison** (D-R)[2]	1751-1836
05	1817-1825	James **Monroe** (D-R)	1758-1831
06	1825-1829	John Quincy **Adams** (R)	1767-1848
07	1829-1837	Andrew **Jackson** (D)	1767-1845
08	1837-1841	Martin **Van Buren** (D)	1782-1862
09	1841	William H. **Harrison** (W)[3]	1773-1841
10	1841-1845	John **Tyler** (W-D)[4]	1790-1862
11	1845-1849	James K. **Polk** (D)	1794-1849
12	1849-1850	Zachary **Taylor** (W)	1784-1850
13	1850-1853	Millard **Fillmore** (W)	1800-1874
14	1853-1857	Franklin **Pierce** (D)	1804-1869
15	1857-1861	James **Buchanan** (D)	1791-1868
16	1861-1865	Abraham **Lincoln** (R)	1809-1865
17	1865-1869	Andrew **Johnson** (R)	1808-1875
18	1869-1877	Ulysses S. **Grant** (R)	1822-1885
19	1877-1881	Rutherford B. **Hayes** (R)	1822-1893
20	1881	James A. **Garfield** (R)	1831-1881
21	1881-1885	Chester A. **Arthur** (R)	1830-1886
22	1885-1889	Grover **Cleveland** (D)	1837-1908
23	1889-1893	Benjamin **Harrison** (R)	1833-1901
24	1893-1897	Grover **Cleveland** (D)	1837-1908
25	1897-1901	William **McKinley** (R)	1843-1901

[1]**Fed**: Federalist; [2]**D-R**: Forerunner of Democratic Party;
[3]**W**: Whig; [4]**W-D**: Ran on Whig ticket but was a Democrat

U.S. Presidents 1901-2001
(26th through 43rd)

No.	Term of Office	President	Life Span
26	1901-1908	Theodore **Roosevelt** (R)	1858-1919
27	1909-1913	William Howard **Taft** (R)	1857-1930
28	1913-1921	Woodrow **Wilson** (D)	1856-1924
29	1921-1923	Warren **Harding** (R)	1865-1923
30	1923-1929	Calvin **Coolidge** (R)	1873-1933
31	1929-1933	Herbert **Hoover** (R)	1874-1964
32	1933-1945	Franklin D. **Roosevelt** (D)	1882-1945
33	1945-1953	Harry S. **Truman** (D)	1884-1972
34	1953-1961	Dwight D. **Eisenhower** (R)	1890-1969
35	1961-1963	John F. **Kennedy** (D)	1917-1963
36	1963-1969	Lyndon B. **Johnson** (D)	1908-1973
37	1969-1974	Richard M. **Nixon** (R)	1913-1994
38	1974-1976	Gerald R. **Ford** (R)	1913-20--
39	1976-1980	James E. **Carter** (D)	1923-20--
40	1980-1992	Ronald **Reagan** (R)	1911-20--
41	1989-1992	George H. **Bush** (R)	1924-20--
42	1992-2000	William J. **Clinton** (D)	1946-20--
43	2000-	George W. **Bush** (R)	1946-20--

To Those Who Go Before Us

Alzheimer's disease is no respecter of persons. It strikes men and women of all nations, famous and unknown, rich and poor, educated and illiterate. Perhaps the most widely recognized individuals standing strong against this dread disease are former President Ronald Reagan and his family. Their forthrightness, bravery, and compassion reassure other AD families that we are not alone, and give us courage to live another day. Thank you, President and Mrs. Reagan.

Presidents' Day
(Third Monday in February)

For a listing of U.S. presidents, refer to pages 140 and 141. This information has been included to help you understand and converse more easily with older impaired family members who may recall presidents and their eras, with which you may not be familiar.

☐ Display an American flag.

☐ Discuss the life of a president you remember or enjoyed reading about.

☐ Look at a picture book of all U.S. presidents. **Caregiver**: If you don't have such a book, borrow one from the library.

☐ Make a presidential collage. **Caregiver**: Help your AD family member paint or color a photocopy of a favorite president, or use a picture from a child's coloring book of presidents. Paste the picture to a larger sheet of construction paper and create a red, white and blue border design with paints, felt-tipped pens, multistriped ribbon, glitter, or other craft materials.

☐ Play a game based on U.S. presidents.

☐ Read a short story or children's book about your favorite president. **Caregiver**: Your local library will have biographies, stories and children's books about individual presidents.

☐ Talk about early school days. What presidents

did you learn about? Which presidents' pictures hung on the classroom wall. (Pictures of Washington and Lincoln were popular.)
❏Watch a video about a U.S. president.

Puzzles

Puzzles can be great fun if they have an appropriate number of pieces for your AD family member's skill level and are presented without pressure for perfection. Be prepared to lend a hand, hint, or encouraging word if needed. Following are several puzzles that can be found in stores and online.

❏Discover cardboard shape puzzles — animals, cars, emergency vehicles, United States map.
❏Enjoy an easy-grip wood puzzle. **Caregiver**: Puzzles with finger-tip grasp knobs and an identical picture underneath each piece make matching pieces easier. Six to nine pieces per puzzle. Men especially enjoy those from Fred Levine Productions featuring tools, construction vehicles, and other vehicles used for transportation and work. $10.95 each.
❏Put together a children's jigsaw puzzle (12-100 pieces). **Caregiver**: Many easy-to-do puzzles are available beginning at around $1.50. Several of the many picture choices should appeal to your A.D. patient or family member.
❏Rediscover word search/word find books. **Care-**

giver: Buy children's word books to make searching easier for your AD family member.
☐Relax with same-and-opposite puzzles. **Caregiver**: Buy books or cards, or make your own cards by cutting in half medium- to large-sized pictures from magazines and gluing each half to a separate sheet of paper.

Radios

Many older people have vivid memories of the early days of radio. As a new invention, it became a popular source of home entertainment during the 1920s and beyond with family members gathered together to listen to favorite programs. President Warren G. Harding was the first U.S. president to speak over the air, at the Minnesota State Fair in September 1920.

☐Discuss favorite old radio programs — news, soap operas, comedies, dramas, mysteries, musical varieties.
☐Listen to audiotapes or CDs of old radio programs. **Caregiver**: You'll find tapes and CDs in music, drug and variety stores, and in many libraries.
☐Visit the library and borrow a book on radio history. **Caregiver**: Select a book with lots of pictures that may refresh memories.
☐Talk about famous people or reported events heard over the radio — the Hindenburg Disas-

ter; newscaster Gabriel Heater; ventriloquist Edgar Bergen with Charlie McCarthy; Ozzie and Harriett; Your Hit Parade; President Franklin D. Roosevelt, or others.
❒Talk about family life during the radio era. What brand was your family's first radio? What did it look like? Who decided what programs to listen to? What other things did you do while listening to the radio? (Knit, sew, iron, smoke a pipe, work a puzzle, do schoolwork, draw?)

Recitation

For older generations of Americans, memorization and learning to recite "by heart" were key elements in their education. More than a few caregivers have been surprised by the number of childhood memorizations their AD family members have retained.

❒Listen to a child recite a memory verse for you.
❒Read a book of favorite old poetry or children's nursery rhymes. **Caregiver**: Encourage your AD family member to recite verses he or she remembers. Assist with forgotten words as needed.
❒Recite a Bible verse.
❒Record your memorized pieces on audio- or videotape.
❒Share a poem you remember with a child.

❏Sing a song you remember from bygone years.
❏Talk about memorizing. What things were you required to memorize when you were a child? What was the longest piece you memorized? Did you recite in front of groups of people — school or church programs, at home, for civic organizations, in contests? Did you receive awards or prizes for excellent recitations?

> *"Aunt Florence can't remember what happened this morning, but she proudly recites a six stanza poem she learned in school seventy-five years ago."*

Reminiscing

This is a quiet, reassuring activity that draws upon your AD family member's earlier life interests, natural abilities and skills. While recalling bygone days, activities, and accomplishments, positive feelings of self-worth are generated. The value of his or her life — past and present — is reaffirmed.

❏Browse through a box of personal keepsakes.
❏Describe your profession or lifetime work to a family member or friend.
❏Listen to favorite old music. **Caregiver**: Play audiotapes, CDs, or let your family member select favorites from a collection of 78 or 45 rpm records.

☐Read or listen to a story about the town or area in which you grew up. **Caregiver**: Contact local historical societies for newsletters containing first person stories and books on local history.

☐Leaf through favorite recipe books.

☐Look at family photographs.

☐Look through school yearbooks. Read the autographs.

☐Rediscover the contents of a family trunk or cedar chest.

☐Share a story about a sports trophy, photo or memory that is important to you.

☐View home movies, videos, slides.

☐Visit or drive by your old family home.

☐Walk down a street where you lived long ago.

The Roaring Twenties

The 1920s were wild years: jazz, the "lost generation," liberated working women, hemlines at the knees, bobbed hair, the Charleston, dance marathons, Prohibition, bootleggers, speakeasies, hip flasks of hooch, smoking, sensuality, gangsters, skyrocketing Wall Street investments (on paper, anyway), Babe Ruth, Knute Rockne, F. Scott Fitzgerald, Charlie Chaplin, Florenz Ziegfeld, the Scopes "monkey" trial, and so much more. Most people who experienced this liberal generation remember it.

☐Bob your hair. (Usually, this is more appealing

to ladies.)

☐ Dance the Charleston.

☐ Listen to music from the 1920s.

☐ Play a game that was popular in the 1920s — checkers, dominoes, Mah Jongg.

☐ Read a selection from *Collected Poems* by Edwin Arlington Robinson, or *So Big* by Edna Ferber.

☐ Reminisce about famous sports figures of the 1920s — Babe Ruth, Jack Dempsey, Lou Gehrig, Red Grange, Rogers Hornsby, Bobby Jones, Bill Tilden. Did you meet or see these or other famous athletes?

☐ Sing a song from the 1920s — *Yes Sir, That's My Baby*, *Happy Days Are Here Again*, *If You Knew Susie (Like I Know Susie)*, *Bye Bye Blackbird*, *My Blue Heaven*, or others.

☐ Talk about your memories of the Roaring 20s. How old were you? Where did you live? What activities were you involved in — school, work, military, other? Did you live in the country or the city? What kind of car did you or your family drive? What were favorite family activities? Was your family for or against Prohibition? Do you remember any funny stories about Prohibition? What was the most exciting thing you did in the '20s?

☐ Visit a museum and view 1920s artifacts.

☐ Watch a television documentary about the '20s.

☐ Watch a videotaped silent film from the 1920s.

☐Watch a video with a 1920s theme. **Caregiver**: Select an upbeat comedy or musical, not a violent gangster film.

> *"During Prohibition, my daddy decided to make beer for the first time. Apparently he did something wrong because one night the bottles began exploding in our basement, scaring our family half to death."*

Rosh Hashanah (Date varies)
The ten days beginning with Rosh Hashanah and ending with Yom Kippur are known as the Days of Awe.

Rosh Hashanah translates to "head" of the year and is New Year's Day in the Jewish calendar. On this day Almighty God opens the Book of Life, an awesome event. It is a solemn but also joyous occasion when Jews renew their acceptance and proclamation of God's Kingship of the Universe and each individual. They repent of their sins and recommit themselves to God, to lead their lives in accordance with His will. They also seek reconciliation with any person they may have wronged during the past year. Rosh Hashanah usually occurs in September. Ten days later, on Yom Kippur, the Book of Life is closed until the following year.

☐Attend religious services.

☐Eat an apple dipped in honey and pray the traditional prayer praising God and asking for His blessing during the new year.

☐Eat special foods that symbolize blessing — the

head of a fish, a pomegranate, *tzimmes*.

❏Eat sweets — *classic honey cake, tzimmes* — so the new year will be as sweet as honey.

❏Go to the synagogue to hear the *shofar* blown.

❏Greet someone with *L'shana tovah*, a shortened form for "May you be inscribed and sealed for a sweet and good year!")

❏Greet someone with "May your name be written in the Book of Life."

❏Help light traditional candles.

❏Help prepare special foods and sweets prior to Rosh Hashanah.

❏Listen to and meditate on readings from the *Torah*.

❏Recite the special *Tashlich* Prayer on the first day of Rosh Hashanah, or on the second day if the first falls on *Shabbat*. **Caregiver**: This is customarily done over a body of flowing water that has fish (Water symbolizes kindness; fish, an ever open eye.) *Tashlich* means to throw away, and past sins and transgressions are symbolically thrown into the water.

❏Recite traditional blessings.

❏Tell a Rosh Hashanah story to a child.

(*also see activities under* **Yom Kippur**)

> "Blessed is he whose help is the God of Jacob,
> whose hope is in the Lord his God,
> the Maker of heaven and earth, the sea,
> and everything in them —
> the Lord, who remains faithful forever."
> —Psalm 146:5-6

Saint Patrick's Day
(March 17)

This is Ireland's greatest national holiday and it is also a holy day. The date commemorates the anniversary of the death of Saint Patrick, the missionary who is the patron saint of Ireland. Because so many Irish men, women and children immigrated to America, Saint Patrick's Day became a popular holiday here, too. Today, most everyone celebrates Saint Patrick's special day — whether they're Irish or not.

☐ Attend mass or other religious service.

☐ Bake Irish soda bread.

☐ Buy a shamrock plant. **Caregiver**: Grocery and variety stores usually carry small, inexpensive plants in March.

☐ Call a couple of people and wish them a happy Saint Patrick's Day.

☐ Color a small bowl of sugar green by stirring in a drop of green food coloring.

☐ Create a floral centerpiece using live or synthetic shamrocks and live or silk spring flowers.

☐ Decorate with preprinted or hand-drawn cutouts of Saint Patrick, shamrocks, leprechauns, top hats, tobacco pipes, the Blarney Stone, or maps of Ireland.

☐ Eat corned beef and cabbage.

☐ Give someone who is not wearing green a shamrock to pin on his or her collar.

☐Listen to traditional Irish music.

☐Pinch someone who is not wearing green.

☐Read a story about Saint Patrick or Ireland.

☐Recite a poem about Saint Patrick or Ireland.

☐Say a special prayer.

☐Share happy stories about Saint Patrick's Day celebrations in your family. Did your extended family gather together? What were your favorite Irish foods, activities and traditions?

☐Talk about your Irish heritage. What was life in America like for your Irish immigrant ancestors? Where did they settle? What was their home like? How many children did they have? What type work did they do in Ireland; in America?

☐Tint carnations green by adding green food coloring to the vase of water the night before.

☐Watch a video featuring Irish dancing such as Riverdance.

☐Wear something green — an article of clothing, a bow in your hair, or a shamrock on your collar or tie.

> "May the road rise to meet you, may the wind be always at your back, the sun shine warm upon your face, the rain fall soft upon your fields, and until we meet again, may God hold you in the palm of His hand. "
>
> —Irish Blessing

School Days

School days, school days,
Good old golden rule days.
Readin' and writin' and 'rithmetic,
Taught to the tune of a hick'ry stick . . .

—popular old song

❑Describe your first day of school. How old were you? What did you wear? Did you feel excited or fearful? Did you go to school alone or with siblings? How did you get to school — walk, ride a bike, travel in a car, ride a horse, take a bus or street car?

❑Recite jump rope rhymes.

❑Sing your high school's or college's official song.

❑Talk about school days. When did you learn to read? Did you learn by the phonics method or some other? What was your grammar school (or high school or college) like — large, small, city, country, public, private, secular, religious? Did you take your lunch to school in a paper bag or lunch box, or did you buy food at school or go home to eat?

❑Watch the movie *Good Morning, Miss Dove* or another film about school days.

"Ninety-year old Maggie never tires of show-ing off her report cards from grammar school and pointing out her excellent grades."

School Yearbooks/Annuals

School yearbooks, once commonly referred to as "annuals," are compiled to preserve photographs of students and events and to commemorate school activities, studies and accomplishments. Browsing through a school yearbook is a little like taking a trip in a time machine. The past comes alive!

☐Browse through old school yearbooks. Look at photos of people and events.

☐Call a high school or college classmate to say hello.

☐Invite a high school or college classmate to visit you.

☐Identify the people in your class photos. **Caregiver**: Record the names for future reference.

☐Look at the photographs of teachers and other adults who worked at your school. Who was your favorite teacher? What do you remember about him or her?

☐Read the autographs in your yearbook.

☐Reminisce about special activities you enjoyed — academic competitions, band or orchestra, choir, clubs, FFA (Future Farmers of America), sports, theatre, or others.

☐Talk about happy memories from that era. Who were your best friends? What did you do together? Did you enjoy school? Classes? Sports? Clubs? How did you get to school? What kind of car did you drive?

Science

Scientific experiments need not be complex to be fun. If you need more challenging projects, you'll find many in books and at online Website resources.

❑Attend a school science fair.

❑Discover televised science programs. **Caregiver**: Choose from Cosmos, Jacques Cousteau, Mr. Wizard's World, National Geographic, Nature, Smithsonian Institution specials, and others. If a science program is too long for your AD family member or patient to watch in one sitting, tape it for later viewing with a VCR.

❑Experiment with magnets. **Caregiver**: Obtain several sizes if possible. Test their positive and negative forces on one another. See how much weight each can hold.

❑Invite a child to share his or her school science project with you.

❑Make bubble fluid and blow bubbles. **Caregiver**: To make fluid, mix 8 tablespoons of dishwashing liquid into 1 quart of water. Pour the fluid into a shallow container. Cut both ends from a tin can (be sure there are no sharp edges), dip one end into the fluid, and blow gently through the other end to form a bubble. It's fun to use small, medium, and large cans to blow bubbles of various sizes. (If you prefer, you can buy plastic bubble-blowing wands at variety and craft stores, or ask children in the family if they will share wands left over from purchased bubble fluid.) This is a great project to enjoy outside on a warm day. The rainbow colors in the bubbles will be more vivid, and the bubbles will float in the breeze.

☐Rediscover "Magic Crystals." **Caregiver**: Magic crystals are available in novelty catalogs, craft stores and online through World of Science. Many of us have fond childhood memories of these colorful crystals that, when put into their special solution, "grow" into a variety of stalagmitic shapes. Around $13 or less.

☐Share a scientific fact or experiment with a child, teenager, family member, or friend.

☐Talk about your career as a scientist. In what field of science did you work? What were your tasks and responsibilities? How old were you when you first became interested in science? Where were you trained for your job — university, on-the-job, technical program? What was your most exciting or important accomplishment? **Caregiver**: Document your AD family member's stories on paper or a tape recorder.

☐Watch a movie about a famous scientist — Marie Curie, Thomas Edison, Albert Einstein, J. Robert Oppenheimer, or others.

Scrapbooks

Old scrapbooks are a joy to browse through, and new scrapbooks provide a failure-free activity that can be added to and enjoyed over a long period of time. Collected items may be pasted in a spiral-bound notebook or inexpensive, hardcover album. Acid-free, archival scrapbook albums designed to last for generations are also available, but they are more expensive and are probably not necessary for your purposes.

☐ Choose a favorite subject to paste in a scrapbook — advertising characters (Campbell Kids, Pillsbury Doughboy, Energizer Rabbit), cartoons, cars, flowers (pictures and pressed), pets, sports, wild animals or others.

☐ Save greeting cards you receive. **Caregiver**: Help your AD family member note the dates the cards arrive and the names of senders. When cards are associated with a party, include photos taken at the celebration, napkins, and samples of giftwrapping, perhaps cut in the shape of a heart. Add sparkle to the page with a sprinkling of colorful confetti or glitter.

☐ Look at and discuss your old scrapbooks. How old were you when you collected these souvenirs? Which souvenirs do you like best? Please share a happy memory about this souvenir. This is an interesting program. . . . Did you go to football games frequently?

☐ Shop for specialty items to add to your scrapbook materials. **Caregiver**: Many stores carry a variety of scrapbook-enhancing products — colorful background papers and borders, templates, photo frames, captions, stickers, how-to books, gel pens, fancy-cut scissors, cutting mats, glitter, and much more.

☐Start a postcard scrapbook. Which postcards prompt pleasant recollections? **Caregiver**: Add titles beneath each postcard for easy identification. Buy new cards or visit secondhand stores and yard sales for old postcards.

Seasonal Activities

Every season becomes a favorite when life is filled with worthwhile and pleasurable happenings for you and your AD family member.

Spring

☐Attach a suction-cup bird feeder to the outside of a window so you can sit in a comfortable chair inside and watch birds eat.

☐Beat dust from rugs.

☐Clean window screens.

☐Create a collage of spring pictures.

☐Drive through the country and look at green hills, surging rivers, creeks, and waterfalls.

☐Fill bird feeders.

☐Go to a major league baseball, spring training

game in Arizona or Florida.

❑Install a two-way thermometer on a window so you can monitor the temperature indoors and out.

❑Pick spring flowers and put them in a water-filled vase.

❑Put a spring-themed tablecloth on the table — flowers, birds, butterflies.

❑Sweep decks, porches, walkways.

❑Visit a farm and watch lambs and colts frolic.

❑Wash windows.

❑Watch for the arrival of spring birds and the sprouting and blooming of spring plants.

❑Work in the garden.

Summer

❑Attend a horseshoe pitching tournament.

❑Attend a swimming meet.

❑Attend an inline skating demonstration or competition.

❑Churn ice cream.

❑Create a collage of summer pictures.

❑Go camping.

❑Go fishing.

❑Hike along a short, easy, picturesque trail.

❑Listen to music at an outdoor concert.

❑Make lemonade or iced tea.

❑Paint a fence.

❑Picnic in the park or backyard.

❑Pitch horseshoes.

☐Put a summer-themed tablecloth on the table —
   beaches, barbecues, patriotic.

☐Relax at a baseball or softball game.

☐Set out ingredients for ice cream sundaes.

☐Toss or roll a beach ball back and forth.

☐Visit a skateboard park and watch the action.

☐Walk to nearby stores.

☐Watch skaters at a roller rink.

☐Water plants.

Fall

☐Clean out gutters.

☐Create a collage of fall pictures.

☐Gather seeds from flowers that have finished
   blooming.

☐Go to a football game.

☐Plant bulbs for spring blooms.

☐Put a fall-themed tablecloth on the table —
   autumn leaves, squirrels gathering nuts, fall
   colors.

☐Put summer clothes in a trunk.

☐Store window screens.

☐Rake and pile fallen leaves.

☐Roast marshmallows and hot dogs in a campfire.

☐Stack firewood for winter use.

Winter

☐Build a snowman.

☐Create a collage of winter pictures.

☐Go to a basketball game.

☐Make candy; pull taffy.

☐Organize boots and mittens.

☐Put a winter-themed tablecloth on the table — ice skaters, snowflakes, winter birds or other cold weather scenes.

☐Shovel snow.

☐Sit by a warm fireplace or heater and sip hot chocolate or cider.

☐Travel to a warm locale for a holiday.

☐Visit a ski area, sit in a warm lodge with big windows, and watch skiers.

☐Watch ice skaters or an ice hockey game at an indoor or outdoor rink.

☐Watch snow fall. Use a magnifying glass to look at snowflakes. Like people, each is wonderfully unique.

Sensory Experiences

You may help keep your AD family member's senses sharper by pleasantly stimulating them with familiar objects. If you make a game of it, all the better. To help relax, reward and reassure, schedule occasional or regular VIP treatments — for your AD family member **and for yourself.**

☐Cream your hands with lotion and wrap them in a moist, heated towel. **Caregiver**: A fluffy, damp hand or bath towel is easy to heat in a microwave oven. Be sure the towel is very warm but not too hot when applied to hands. Massaging the hands and fingers is a bonus treatment.

☐Feel objects in a bag and guess what each is without looking at it. **Caregiver**: A soft, velvety bag is ideal for this activity, but if you don't want to buy or make one, use a plastic or paper bag. Place a few familiar objects of varying shapes and textures in the bag — spoon, comb, brush, ball of yarn, paper clips, leather wallet, coins, sandpaper, emery board, cotton ball, wrapped candies, etc. Give helpful hints if your AD family member needs them. Take turns, encouraging your AD family member to select objects for you to guess.

☐Have a facial.

☐Have a manicure or pedicure.

☐Have a hand, foot, shoulder, or full-body massage.

☐Massage your feet, back or shoulders with electric vibrating massagers.

☐Scratch your back with a hand-held scratcher.

☐Splash or spray on after-shave or perfume.

☐Soak your feet in a warm footbath.

☐Soften your hands and face with lotion.

☐Visit a beauty salon or barber shop for a haircut or perm.

"Some patients who were agitated calmed down when we patted their backs or gently

massaged their shoulders. There seems to be something almost magical in the human touch."

TIP: If your AD family member's hands are cold, warm a damp towel in the microwave and wrap it around his or her hands. Be sure the towel is warm, not hot. Rewarm the towel when it cools down.

Service Clubs/Civic Organizations

If you are a caregiver for a man or woman who was a member of a service club or civic organization, show your appreciation for their contributions to community improvement projects. Clubs and organizations include but are not limited to the following: American Association for Retired Persons (AARP), Chamber of Commerce, Grange, Junior League, Kiwanis, Lions, Masonic Lodge, International Order of Oddfellows (IOOF), Optimists, Parent Teacher Association (PTA), Rotary, Soroptimists, Veterans of Foreign Wars (VFW).

❑Attend a parade in which your service club will be participating. Wave to members as they pass by.
❑Talk about your service club. Which club did you (or do you) belong to? Why did you decide to join this club? Who was your best

friend in the club?

☐Talk about your service club projects. What projects did you participate in? Were you in charge of any projects? What was your favorite project? What was the biggest project your club undertook?

Sewing Room

Stitching doesn't have to be perfect to be pleasurable, and many men will enjoy some of the following activities, too.

> **WARNING:** Before planning activities in which a potentially dangerous device such as an iron, sewing machine, or sharp implement will be used, <u>make sure your family member is capable of safely working with it.</u>

☐Fold fabric.

☐Iron fabric.

☐Separate embroidery thread into small plastic bags.

☐Sort button sets into egg cartons or bags.

☐Select and sort fabric for quilt blocks or other sewing projects.

☐Sharpen scissors.

☐Undo half-knitted or crocheted projects.

☐Wind yarn into balls.

☐Make potholders or other simple projects on small, hand-held weaving looms.
☐Stitch quilt blocks by hand or with a sewing machine.

> When planning activities remember **K I S S**.
> **Keep It Simple, Sweetheart!**

Shopping

Shopping together can be great fun for you and your AD family member, but do not shop 'til you drop. Allow enough time for shopping so you are not rushed, and sit down or call it a day as soon as the first hint of exhaustion begins to occur.

☐Browse in a favorite store or specialty shop.
☐Buy a gift for someone special.
☐Create a shopping collage using pictures of favorite "purchases" cut from magazines or catalogs and pasted onto construction paper. **Caregiver**: Narrow subject matter by selecting pictures for a kitchen, bedroom, bathroom, yard, etc.
☐Make a list of things you want to look at or buy at the store.
☐Visit a candy store and choose favorite chocolates. Talk about favorite childhood candies. What was your favorite candy when

you were a child? How much did candy cost then? Did you, your mother or grandmother make candy? Were you allowed to eat candy every day or only at special events?

❏Stroll in an enclosed shopping mall during winter storms or summer heat.

Sorting/Matching

A sorting activity may serve a practical purpose or simply be an enjoyable game. Your AD family member or patient may enjoy a variety of sorting activities or prefer to sort the same objects repeatedly. The important thing is to choose objects that can be easily sorted. Be helpful and patient, and don't worry if the end result isn't perfect. The following activities and suggestions have proved successful.

❏Pair objects — socks, mittens, gloves, baby shoes, earrings.

❏Enjoy *Playful Patterns*, matching basic shapes to patterns on cards. **Caregiver**: Patterns progress from very simple to moderately complex. The shaped pieces are colorful and texturally appealing. If your loved one is not able to match the pieces easily, make a game of it and take turns. $17.99. Discovery Toys.

❏Sort family photos. **Caregiver**: Help your AD family member match husbands with wives, children with parents, brothers with sisters, grandparents with grandchildren. Photocopy or computer scan photos and glue onto cards. Laminate for durability.

❑Sort household objects by category — candles, corks, coupons, hair clips, paper clips, pot holders, rubber bands, jar lids, spice containers, spoons, thimbles, thread spools.

❑Sort with a deck of handcrafted sorting cards. **Caregiver**: A set of 56 cards is standard but sets with fewer cards work well, too. For simplicity, use colors or basic shapes on heavyweight paper. Add variety later if it is appropriate. Laminate cards for durability.

❑Sort with purchased decks of sorting cards and sorting games. **Caregiver**: You'll find sorting cards in educational, variety, and toy stores, or order them through the Super Duper Publications catalog. Prices vary.

❑Sort toy objects by category. **Caregiver**: Choose a few small, easy-to-handle, unbreakable toys — airplanes, animals, babies, birds, blocks, butterflies, canned food, cars, clothing, dishes, dolls, fruit, furniture, people, tools, train cars, trucks, vegetables.

❑Sort objects by size — small, medium, large.

❑Sort objects by color. **Caregiver**: Use a deck of colored cards, crayons, wood blocks, fabric or felt swatches, felt-tipped pens, marbles, plastic Easter eggs, sheets of paper.

☐Sort objects by patterns. **Caregiver**: Use cards or sheets of paper with horizontal stripes, vertical stripes, wavy lines, dots, circles, squares, or other designs.

☐Sort things that go together: apple/tree; baby/ mother; bird/birdhouse; ball/bat; cake/ candles; Christmas tree/ornament; Easter egg/ basket; egg/hen; fish/bowl; flower/watering can; foot/shoe; hand/mitten; moon/stars.

> **TIP:** Sort small objects into plastic ice cube trays, egg cartons, or divided boxes. Sort medium and larger items into margarine tubs or other containers.

Spanish American War (1898)

This 1898 war between the United States and Spain occurred more than 100 years ago when President William McKinley was in office, so few people living today will remember it. However, history buffs may know facts about it, and others may remember stories their parents or grandparents told about this well-publicized event that captured newspaper headlines across the nation. The war began after the U.S. battleship Maine exploded in Havana harbor, killing 260 men. Those responsible for the explosion were never officially identified. After the attack on the Maine, the U.S. joined Cuba in its revolt against Spain.

☐Look through a historical picture book about the Spanish American War.

❑Read a book or story about the Spanish American War or a famous American who lived during that era. **Caregiver**: Easy-to-read children's books found at the library are ideal for the AD patient with a limited attention span.

❑Talk about famous men and women who lived during the Spanish American War era — President William McKinley, political leader/orator William Jennings Bryan, newspaper publisher William Randolph Hearst, author Booth Tarkington, or others. Did you learn about any of these people in school? Do you recall why they were famous?

❑Talk about your family's memories and stories of the Spanish American War. In what states did your ancestors live during that period of history? Did men in your family fight in this war?

❑Visit a memorial or museum and look at artifacts from the Spanish American War.

Spiritual

"The Spirit of God has made me;
the breath of the Almighty gives me life."
—Job 33:4

❑Attend church or other religious services.
❑Attend religious holiday programs, especially

musical events that include children, skits, or other movement.

☐Invite a child to share his or her favorite Bible story or memory verse with you.

☐Keep a prayer journal to list people and things you pray for and prayers answered. **Caregiver**: If you need to help your AD family member with writing prayer requests in the journal, make them as simple as possible — good health for John, sunshine for Ruth's wedding, completion of noisy construction next door. Journals with blank pages are readily available at a variety of prices, or use an inexpensive spiral-bound notebook. Decorate the cover and include colorful stickers on the inside pages.

☐Listen to a sermon or spiritual service on the radio or on an audiotape.

☐Listen to spiritual music.

☐Make a "blessing book" to list things you are grateful for. **Caregiver**: If your AD family member needs help, write down blessings as he or she dictates them. In the beginning, you may also need to suggest blessings — a warm sweater, flowers in bloom, a pet, a letter, etc. (See "prayer journal" above for information on types of journals.) Review the blessings in life frequently.

☐Pray and meditate in a "placid place" reserved especially for that purpose. **Caregiver**: The placid place can be as simple as a rose-covered arbor in the garden or a comfortable chair in a quiet corner of the house.

☐Read brief daily devotionals.

☐Read and talk about the *Bible* or simple *Bible* stories together. What is your favorite *Bible* story? Who is your favorite person in the *Bible*? Would you like to have lived during *Bible* times?

☐Read inspirational books and poetry.

☐Recite scripture or inspirational verses memorized long ago.

☐Serve as a church greeter.

☐Sing favorite spiritual songs.

☐Visit with spiritually like-minded friends.

Caregiver: Request regular visits from members of local religious congregations.

☐Watch a movie with a spiritual theme.

☐Watch a religious service on television.

Sports

Old athletic skills, physical prowess, and the competitive edge may be lost to your AD family member, but if his or her love of sporting events remains, rekindle team spirit with win-win activities.

☐Collect sports figurines.

☐Collect trading cards of your favorite sport.

☐Collect sports memorabilia in a scrapbook — pictures of athletes, game tickets, newspaper and magazine articles, programs, miniature banners, etc.

☐Go to a ball game, major or minor league or local. **Caregiver**: Enjoy the game with your family member. Eat hot dogs, popcorn and big, soft pretzels. For outdoor events, wear hats and sunscreen on sunny days or keep warm in parkas and cozy blankets on cold days.

☐Have your picture taken at a sporting event. **Caregiver**: Help your AD family member mount the snapshot in an album and note the date and location for later reminiscing.

☐Look through your old sports scrapbooks or the sports sections of your high school or college yearbooks.

☐Make a sports collage. Cut pictures from magazines and glue them on construction paper.

☐Make sports-themed gift wrap paper. Use white or other solid-color paper and decorate it with pictures and headlines cut from sports magazines and newspapers.

☐Talk about your sports career. What was your favorite sport? Where did you play it? How old were you? What positions did you play? What were your most exciting plays and accomplishments? Who were your teammates or best friends on the team? Did you teach others how to play or improve their game?

☐Talk about your sports interests. Which sports do you enjoy? Which are your favorite teams? Favorite players? Who do you think was the best player of all time? Is there a game or event you remember best? Why was it exciting? Who is your favorite sportscaster?

> *"At a summer baseball game, I sat behind a father and son. The older man was afflicted with Alzheimer's disease, and I was deeply touched by the tenderness and patience the son showed him. The old fellow didn't talk at all, but his joy was revealed by his broad smile."*

Star Gazing

Most of us have been "wishing on a star" since we first learned to talk. Take advantage of this natural fascination with the heavens by turning wishful thinking into star-studded activities.

☐Bake star-shaped sugar cookies.
☐Create a nighttime collage. **Caregiver**: Help your AD family member cut out yellow or silver moon and stars (or use stickers). Glue them on black or dark blue construction paper. Use a silver gel pen to design a border and add glitter for drama.
☐Decorate the bedroom ceiling or lamp shade

with glow-in-the-dark stars.

☐Listen to or sing music with a nighttime theme — *Fly Me to the Moon*, *Moonlight Serenade*, *Some Enchanted Evening*, *Stardust*, *That's Amore* ("When the moon hits your eye like a big pizza pie, that's amore . . ."), *When You Wish upon a Star*, and others. Add to your list as other appropriate songs are recalled.

☐Look at the stars and moon on a warm evening.

☐Make a heavenly mobile. **Caregiver**: Buy a kit or start from scratch with a wire clothes hanger, fishing line and sun, moon and stars cutouts. Add glitter for sun- or starshine and moonglow.

☐Make a wish on the evening's first star.

☐Observe a meteor shower, usually forecast in newspapers. **Caregiver**: If the weather is warm, stretch out on patio loungers.

☐Read a simple book or story about a famous star gazer such as Polish astronomer Nicolaus Copernicus.

☐Recite a childhood verse featuring heavenly bodies. **Caregiver**: You can also make a game of this by taking turns reciting half of each rhyme. "Star light, star bright," (. . . first star I see tonight); "Twinkle, twinkle, little star," (. . . how I wonder what you are); "Hey, diddle diddle, the cat and the fiddle," (. . . the cow jumped over the moon) or others.

☐Visit a planetarium.

Story Time

Tape record, videotape, or write down original creative fiction and family stories. This will be especially meaningful to future generations.

☐Make a game of storytelling. **Caregiver**: Take turns inventing a story, with one person beginning the story, another person continuing it, and then switching back and forth (or progressing around a circle of people) until story's end. The sillier the story, the better. Laughter is good medicine.

☐Tell stories frequently. **Caregiver**: Set aside a special time to tell stories — remembered tales from childhood, folklore, or original creations.

> *"During Great-grandma's final years in an Arizona nursing home, a newspaper reporter interviewed her about her childhood on the plains. How I treasure that information!"*

> *"At Christmas, I gave each of my children a booklet of life-experience stories I had transcribed from recordings of interviews with my father. He had lived what he described as a simple life, but to the kids, Papa's adventures as an Illinois cattleman were very exciting."*

☐Tape record stories on a trip. **Caregiver**: Take a

small tape recorder on automobile trips to capture conversations and family stories.

❐ Talk about life experiences. **Caregiver**: Stories from the past are often remarkably full of accurate details, a treasure trove for family historians.

Childhood: What is your earliest memory? Did you have brothers and sisters? Who was older and who younger? What did your father do for a living? What was your home like? Where did you go to grammar school? What were your grandparents (or other relatives) like? Do you look like your mother or father?

Teens: What type clothes did you wear? What music/musician was popular? What type car did you drive? Where did you go on dates? Did you have a job? What did you do with money earned? Did you enjoy sports? Which ones? Did you ever play any practical jokes or pranks during your teens?

Adult: Did you go to college? What type job did you have? Where or how were you trained to do your job? How many years did you work there? How did you meet your spouse? How old were you when you got married? What was your wedding like? How many children do you have? What are their names? What did you do in your spare time?

❐ Visit a street or town where you grew up or lived and describe your life there.

Telephones

On March 7, 1876, the first U.S. patent for the telephone was issued to Alexander Graham Bell, and by 1878 there were 10,755 telephones in service. Life without telephones is unimaginable today, but in bygone eras, not every American family had a phone. Some lived in areas too rural for such sophisticated devices; others used neighbors' telephones for emergencies. Whatever their personal telephone history, all older Americans have seen many changes in telephone styles and applications. Telephone activities that tap into past and present experiences help maintain open lines of communication with AD family members.

❑Enjoy frequent calls from family and friends. **Caregiver**: You may need to encourage, request, and schedule regular calls from family members and close friends. Also consider calling your church or senior center and if they have telephone visiting services, schedule a regular call for your loved one.

❑Call friends and relatives. **Caregiver**: Help your loved one dial the phone and regularly connect with the outside world.

❑Talk about your telephone experiences. Did your family have a telephone when you were a child? What was it like? Did you ever use or see a hand-cranked telephone? How did you make long-distance calls? Do you know anyone who was a telephone operator?

❑Watch a movie or documentary about Alexander Graham Bell.

Telephone Timeline Snapshot

1876 — Alexander Graham Bell invents the telephone and receives a U.S. patent for it the same year. Bell's electromagnetic transmitter is also used as the receiver. The user moves the device to the ear to hear and to the mouth to speak.

1877 — Commercial telephone service, Bell Telephone Company, is established.

1878 — First wall telephone. The bulk of the telephone hangs on the wall, and the earpiece is separate.

1878 — First commercial switchboard, New Haven, Connecticut. Using a hand crank, a caller signals a telephone operator to request a specific number. The operator then connects the lines at the switchboard.

1878 — First telephone in the White House, for President Rutherford B. Hayes.

1880s — First desk telephone. The transmitter is also the receiver. The telephone is attached to a large box containing the ringer and, in some cases, the magneto.

1881 — First public U.S. long-distance line, between Boston, Massachusetts and Providence, Rhode Island.

1890 — First international phone line, between Detroit, Michigan and Windsor, Ontario.

1891 — Automatic telephone dialing system is patented.

1891 — Public coin telephones are introduced.

1892 — The desk telephone mouthpiece and headset are combined, but the phone is still attached to a big box containing the ringer and, sometimes, the magneto.

1915 — First long distance line between New York and San Francisco.

1920s — Dial telephones become practical.

1927 — First commercial telephone service by radio, between New York and London.

1930s — First desk phones with ringer, network and handset in one unit.

1950s — First color telephones introduced using cradle phone designs from the 1920s and 1930s.

1960s — Princess phone, Trimline and myriad other telephone designs with varying functions become available.

1980s — First cellular telephones.

1990s — First computerized telephones.

—Various Sources

Television

Television can be a real blessing to families caring for Alzheimer's patients. Most will sit contentedly watching favorite programs, and if you share the activity with them, you have the added benefit of relaxing and conversing about the program. Avoid shows with content that is stressful to your loved one — slow and boring, overtly sexual, violent, and personally distasteful subjects.

> **TIP:** Buy a cordless headphone to help your AD family member adjust TV volume as loud as he or she wants without hurting others' ears and, if he isn't hard of hearing, to focus on the program without distractions. You may have to help turn on and adjust the headphones. About $100 for quality headphones and worth every penny.

❏ Discuss favorite television programs. What do you like about them — the actors, athletes, games, animals, costumes, comedy, stories, action?

❏ Dust the television in preparation for viewing.

❏ Help work a crossword puzzle in a TV program guide.

❏ Invite a friend over to watch a favorite program with you.

❏ Reminisce about your television experiences. When did you watch your first television? What size was the screen? Was the picture black and white or color, clear or snowy? What kind of antenna did your TV have — on the roof, rabbit ears? Did family or friends gather with you to watch shows? Do you recall the first TV shows you saw? Did you eat popcorn, pizza, chips and dip?

❑Select a program to watch. **Caregiver**: To avoid confusion and frustration, offer only a limited number of programing options, perhaps two or three, and describe the contents simply.

❑Talk about television commercials. Which ones do you remember best or were your favorites? Do you recall Ajax, the foaming cleanser; Mr. Clean; the Toni Twins (Which Twin Has the Toni?); Milton Berle's singing Texaco men; Joe Namath in panty hose; Campbell Soup's "Mmm, mmm, good;" the Doublemint Twins; J-E-L-L-O; the Budweiser frogs; Where's the Beef?; the Marlboro Man; the Taco Bell Chihuahuas ("Yo quiero Taco Bell.")?

❑Watch a new program. **Caregiver**: Turn to a show your AD family member has not watched before, perhaps something on science, history, new discoveries, or a game show.

> *"My dad had always enjoyed cops and robbers shows, but after he developed Alzheimer's, these programs gave him terrible nightmares. The problem was solved by selecting nonviolent shows for him."*

Television Timeline Snapshot

1927 — Philo Farnsworth, an American, patents his "dissector tube," a key component in the development of television.

1928 — First TV drama, *The Queen's Messenger* airs from Schenectady, New York.

1939 — NBC debuts at the World's Fair; first baseball game broadcast, NBC.

1947 — *Howdy Doody, Meet the Press* and 15-minute national newscasts air.

1949 — Sears-Roebuck catalog includes television sets.

1951 — *I Love Lucy* starring Lucille Ball and Desi Arnaz premiers.

1953 — *TV Guide* is available at newsstands.

1954 — Senator Joseph McCarthy hearings broadcast live on ABC.

1955 — First presidential news conference is covered by TV, President Eisenhower; *The 64,000 Question* game show airs.

1955-56 — Westerns *Death Valley Days*, *Gunsmoke*, *Tales of the Texas Rangers*, and *Wyatt Earp* air.

1960 — First televised presidential candidate debate, between John F. Kennedy and Richard M. Nixon; *The Flintstones* premiers.

1961 — First live televised presidential press conference, President Kennedy.

1961-62 — Medical dramas *Ben Casey* and *Dr. Kildare* air

1962 — Johnny Carson replaces Jack Paar as *Tonight Show* host.

1964 — First National Football League game broadcast; *Mission Impossible*, *I Spy*, *The Man from U.N.C.L.E.*, and *Get Smart* premier.

1967 — First Super Bowl broadcast; PBS is formed.

1969 — Astronaut Neil Armstrong's moon walk is televised; *Sesame Street* airs.

1971 — *All in the Family* airs.

1973 — Senate Watergate hearings are broadcast live.

1974 — First televised presidential resignation (also first U.S. president to resign), Richard Nixon.

1977 — First television miniseries, *Roots*, airs.

1980s — *The Simpsons*, *ER*, *NYPD Blue*, *Friends* premier.

1990s — *Cheers*, *Dallas*, *Hill Street Blues*, *Love Boat* air

—Various sources

Thanksgiving
(Fourth Thursday in November)

The Pilgrims arrived in the New World in 1620 and struggled through a severe winter in which half of the approximately 100 settlers died. In October 1621 at what is now Plymouth, Massachusetts, the Pilgrims celebrated their survival and blessings, feasting and enjoying games with the native Wampanoags for three days. It was the first Thanksgiving.

☐Arrange a bouquet of fall flowers.

☐Arrange miniature Thanksgiving figures or other decorations on the dining room table.

☐Bake or decorate Thanksgiving cookies.

☐Call a relative or friend and wish him or her a happy Thanksgiving.

☐Count your blessings. **Caregiver**: Help your AD family member if needed. Record blessings in a journal or on a sheet of paper, and read them from time to time.

☐Crack and shell pecans for pecan pie.

☐Fill a bowl with spicy potpourri.

☐Fill a purchased cornucopia with fruits, nuts and vegetables.

☐Fold fruit and nuts into gelatin or whipped cream or nondairy topping.

☐Fold napkins.

☐Gather fall leaves and sprinkle them around the dining table centerpiece.

☐Go for a walk after breakfast or lunch.

☐Greet guests.

☐Help plan the menu.

☐Mix ingredients for the filling of a traditional pumpkin pie.

☐Pose for a picture with family members and friends. **Caregiver**: Help put the snapshot in an album. Record names and date to help recall this special occasion.

☐Place candles in holders and arrange on the table.

☐Put a Thanksgiving or fall-themed tablecloth on the table.

☐Read a story about Thanksgiving.

☐Say a prayer of thanks for your blessings.

☐Send a Thanksgiving Day card to someone special. Decorate the envelope with Thanksgiving stickers or drawings.

☐Serve small cups of eggnog to guests.

☐Set the table.

☐Share a memorable Thanksgiving story with a youngster.

☐Sprinkle nutmeg on cups of eggnog.

☐Stuff celery with soft cheese or peanut butter.

☐Talk about past Thanksgivings. How did your family celebrate when you were a child? Did you traditionally eat at home, with relatives or friends, at a restaurant? What was your favorite part of the meal? What did you do for entertainment — play games, watch television, read, go for a ride? What is your happiest Thanksgiving memory?

❑ Tear up lettuce for a salad.
❑ Thank someone for a compliment, gift, or kindness to you.
❑ Visit with family and friends.
❑ Wash fresh cranberries and pour into a pan to cook into cranberry sauce.
❑ Watch a televised football game.
❑ Watch the annual Macy's Thanksgiving Day parade on television.
❑ Wear a Thanksgiving pin or other jewelry.

Father, We Thank Thee

For health and food, for love and friends,
For everything thy goodness sends,
Father in heaven, we thank Thee.

—Ralph Waldo Emerson

Theatre Arts

Live stage productions and presentations are charged with energy that results from the interaction of performers and audiences. If you have not yet discovered the joy of sharing local performing arts with your AD family member, give it a try.

❑ Attend community theatre productions of fun-filled, popular musicals. **Caregiver**:

Children's productions are often ideal. Some of our family's favorites are *Annie, Charlie's Aunt, Guys and Dolls, The Music Man, Oliver, Peter Pan, Seven Brides for Seven Brothers, The Pajama Game, The Sound of Music, South Pacific, The Wizard of Oz,* and there are many others.

> *"Grandpa Jim, who had never been to a live theatre production, greatly enjoyed seeing his great-granddaughter in* Oliver. *He didn't grasp much of the plot, but he loved the music and dancing and said he wanted to go again."*

❑Discover ethnic instrumentalists and music — African, Celtic, East Indian, Italian, Klezmer, and others. **Caregiver**: Look in the telephone yellow pages for local performers and teachers. Call for performing schedules and locations.

❑Enjoy concerts. **Caregiver**: Watch your newspaper for free community concerts, or plan a night out at a more formal concert hall.

❑Go to a musical instrument competition — accordion, bagpipe, band, banjo, fiddle, guitar, harmonica, harp, piano, ukulele, or other.

❑Relax to a chamber quartet.

❑Reminisce while experiencing music from your youth — blue grass, blues, country, big band, jazz, rock 'n roll, swing. **Caregiver**: Don't overlook one-person presentations at senior centers.

❑Experience an evening at an opera or operetta. **Caregiver**: Check the entertainment section of your newspaper for local as well as big city performances, and select lighthearted productions like those of Gilbert and Sullivan.

❑Listen to poetry at a public reading. **Caregiver**: For lovers of poetry, this is especially pleasant in a small group setting.

❑Schedule an afternoon in the city and take in a matinee performance of a play. **Caregiver**: Select a production that is lighthearted or comedic.

❑Watch amateur and professional dance performances and competitions — ballet, tap, jazz, square dancing. **Caregiver**: Include ethnic dance programs, too — American folk, Greek, Hawaiian, Irish, Israeli, Mexican, Native American, Ukrainian, Scottish, Spanish and others.

> *"Although Elise is often unkempt and disruptive, she eagerly dresses for an evening out and is always on her best behavior in public."*

"The best way out of a difficulty is through it."
—Anonymous

Thrift Shops, Factory Outlets, & Consignment Stores

Everyone enjoys saving money on purchases, and some of the best bargains are to be found at thrift shops, factory outlets, and consignment stores. You and your AD family member will enjoy the time and dollars saved during a trip to one of the following. Allow enough time for leisurely looking.

Thrift Shops

Under the telephone yellow pages listing for "Thrift Shops," you will find contact information on nonprofit businesses managed by Home Hospice, Goodwill Industries, The Salvation Army, St. Vincent de Paul, Y.M.C.A., local church and charitable groups, Welfare League, Veterans Charities, animal welfare organizations, and many others.

❒Shop at charitable stores that carry a wide variety of new and used items, from costume jewelry to furniture and appliances to automobiles.

❒Buy specific new and used items — clothing, furniture, pet supplies, etc. — at shops that specialize.

❒Clean out a drawer or closet and donate items you don't need to a favorite thrift shop. **Caregiver**: Encourage your AD family member to be generous and help others by giving good, resalable items.

"Granny Nivens worried about wasting money at department stores, but she never tired of going to the local Salvation Army Thrift Shop where she bought 'treasures' for pennies."

Factory Outlets

To find retail outlets in your area, look in the telephone yellow pages under specific products — appliances, bakery, clothing, plants, shoes, etc. — or contact the chamber of commerce for a list of local outlets.

❑Discover the variety of low-cost, fresh and day-old breads and pastries at bakery outlet stores.

❑Stock your cupboard at a canned food outlet.

❑Shop for household items at outlets that carry automotive products, dishes, furniture, linens, pots and pans, garden supplies, and numerous other items.

❑Try on and buy all types of garments at clothing outlets — coats, dresses, hats, scarves, shoes, boots, sweaters, and more.

Consignment Stores

Consignment stores are listed in the telephone yellow pages under "Consignment Services." Some consignment stores are in business to make a profit. Others are operated by nonprofit charities. Both offer good deals to customers.

❑Visit an antiques and collectibles consignment

store for an item to add to a favorite collection.

☐ Browse through a consignment clothing store.

☐ Buy a gift for a friend's or relative's youngster at a children's consignment store.

☐ Look for furniture that matches yours at a furniture consignment store.

☐ Sell items you no longer use or wear through a consignment store.

> **"No matter the jargon,**
> **A bargain's a bargain."**
> —Beatrice Gage

Tools

Most men enjoy working with tools, and I was delighted to discover these simple but macho activities. Women are increasingly enjoying tool activities, too, but it still remains mainly Man's domain.

☐ Collect miniature tools.

☐ Discuss tools you have used. Which tool is most useful? How old were you when you learned to use your first tool? Who helped you learn to use tools? What was the most expensive tool you ever used? What was your favorite thing to build with tools? What was the biggest mistake you ever made using a tool?

☐Look through a pictorial book on the history of tools.

☐Put together an easy-grip, wood puzzle of tools (hammer; screwdriver; saw; power drill; wrench; pliers; screws, nuts and bolts; tape measure; level). **Caregiver**: This nine-piece puzzle features finger-tip grasp knobs and an identical picture underneath each puzzle piece to make matching easier. Fred Levine Productions, $10.95.

☐Sort through a box of favorite small tools.

> *"Emil took center stage in front of our group and listed the many tools he had used to build a home. Then he held up a short index finger, chuckled, and said he had cut off its tip with a power saw."*

Tours

Most communities have companies and factories that offer tours of their facilities, free samples, gift shops, and discount thrift stores. Consider the following for your AD family member. Check with your local chamber of commerce or consult the telephone yellow pages for others.

☐Art studio
☐Auto maker
☐Candle factory

☐Candy factory
☐Bakery
☐Cheese factory
☐Coffee mill
☐Farms and ranches
☐Fish hatchery
☐Furniture manufacturer
☐Glass factory
☐Pasta maker
☐Wine Country/Winery

Trains

For many people, trains bring back myriad memories, and your loved one may have wonderful stories to share.

☐Collect miniature train cars and objects associated with trains.
☐Collect picture postcards of trains, and save them in a photo album.
☐Cut pictures of trains from magazines and paste them in a scrapbook. **Caregiver**: If the information is available, include information about the trains for later discussions. Encourage your AD family member to share the scrapbook with a child.
☐Invite a child to read his or her favorite train story to you.
☐Look at a pictorial history book of trains. Did

you ever see any of these trains? What memories do the pictures bring back?

"Cooper recalls that when he was a boy, cattle were herded down the center of town to the railroad depot, where he and many other children gathered to watch the cattle loaded into boxcars."

❒Help set up a model train track.
❒Invite a child to share a train video with you, perhaps one of those featuring Thomas the Tank Engine.
❒Take a train ride. **Caregiver**: Choose a full-sized locomotive or a miniature train at an amusement park.
❒Talk about trains. Did you ever ride on a train? How far did you travel? What sights did you see? Did you enjoy it? Did you ever see a circus train? What were the trains of your childhood like? Did you wave to the engineer or caboose man? What things did the train carry through your town — people, produce, cattle, other products?
❒Tour a train museum.
❒Visit someone who has a train set.
❒Watch a child play with a train set.
❒Watch a movie, video or television program featuring trains — *The Great Train Robbery*, *American Railroads Past and Present* (A&E), *Giants on the Rails*, or others.

Travel

Most caregivers skillfully manage short, routine auto-mobile trips with their AD family members, but few are willing to tackle an extensive trip or a vacation away from home with an AD patient. Some do, however, and enjoy the journey. If your AD family member is not too difficult to manage and you plan ahead carefully, you and your loved one may find the break in the usual routine a joyous, freeing experience.

☐Collect picture postcards of places you visit.

☐Enjoy a day trip to visit a relative or friend. **Caregiver**: Pick a destination you can easily drive to and return from in a day or less, allowing for rest stops along the way. Buy a legally compliant, moveable sun screen to soften harsh glare through windows. Dress comfortably, and take along pillows and a lap robe or extra wrap for your AD family member's comfort. Prepare snacks to nibble on along the way. Enjoy lunch in a restaurant or pack a picnic lunch to eat at a roadside rest stop.

> "Visits should be short, like a winter's day,
> Lest you're too troublesome, hasten away."
> —Benjamin Franklin, 1733

☐Go to a family reunion. **Caregiver**: Relatives will appreciate the stories based on long-term memories of kinfolk and past family events.

☐Create a scrapbook of souvenirs from your travels. **Caregiver**: Document names, dates, locations and interesting facts about the sights or trips.

☐Pose for a snapshot on your trip. **Caregiver**: Help your AD family member mount the photo in an album and note the date and location.

☐Visit a popular scenic destination and spend the night. **Caregiver**: Within a one day's drive of your home, you are likely to find a variety of beautiful spots — daffodil meadows, blooming cherry trees, forests, lakes, rivers, seashores, prairie vistas, painted deserts, snow-capped mountains, orchards, ranches, vineyards, waterfalls, or others.

☐Take a short trip by air, boat or train, just for the experience.

☐Travel to a distant vacation spot and spend a week or two. **Caregiver**: Make a check list and pack supplies to meet your AD family member's needs — clothing, hats, special foods, medications, vitamins, incontinence pads, favorite pillow, books, games, etc.

> "He has put his angels in charge of you to watch over you wherever you go."
> —Psalm 91:11

United Nations Day
(October 24)

This special day commemorates the founding of the United Nations. Through it, people worldwide learn about the United Nations' aim, purposes and achievements. The organization's name was coined by President Franklin D. Roosevelt and was first officially used in January 1942 when 26 nations pledged to fight together against the Axis Powers of World War II.

☐Collect miniature flags of other countries.

☐Discuss one or more of the member countries in the United Nations. **Caregiver**: Help your AD family member find the country on a map or world globe.

☐Browse through a catalog of gifts and publications available through the United Nations Bookstore.

☐Look through a picture book of nations' flags. Which one do you like best?

☐Play a card game that originated in another part of the world.

☐Read a story about the United Nations.

☐View a movie that is set in a foreign country.

☐Watch a documentary on the evolution of the United Nations.

> Alzheimer's disease, a vile terrorist that attacks men and women of all nations, will one day be captured and eliminated. —Anonymous

Valentine's Day
(February 14)

The exact origin of this holiday is uncertain, but its source is thought to have been the ancient Roman festival of Lupercalia, a fertility festival held on February 15. After the Romans became Christian, church leaders decided to Christianize the holiday. They adopted February 14 as the official date, the anniversary of the day a martyred Roman priest, Valentine, was made a saint. For hundreds of years on February 14, people have been sending tokens of affection to those they love.

☐ Bake and decorate heart-shaped cookies or cake.

☐ Buy Valentine's cards in a store or through a catalog.

☐ Call someone you love.

☐ Create home-crafted Valentine's cards.

☐ Cut out pink and red hearts for Valentine's decorations.

☐ Decorate exterior of Valentine's envelopes with hearts and flowers.

☐ Dress for the day in red or pink, hearts and flowers.

☐ Fill a bowl with Valentine's candies.

☐ Insert heart-shaped candies, decorative stickers, or gift enclosures in Valentine's cards.

☐ Insert cards into envelopes and seal them.

☐ Learn to say "I love you" in American Sign Language (ASL).

☐Make and decorate heart-shaped Jell-O. **Caregiver**: Use red Jell-O and garnish with whipped cream and pink and red sprinkles or maraschino cherries and chopped nuts.
☐Pin a Valentine on your collar.
☐Sign Valentine's cards or use a rubber stamp to add your signature.

Veterans Day (Fourth Monday in October, formerly November 11)

Originally called "Armistice Day," this holiday commemorated the end of the fighting in World War I on November 11, 1918. In 1954 President Dwight D. Eisenhower proclaimed the new name, "Veteran's Day," to honor the dead of all wars. The Veterans Day symbol is the red poppy, from the poem "In Flanders' Fields" by Canadian John McCrae, who fought and died in Belgium during World War I.

☐Arrange a bouquet of red poppies.
☐Attend a religious or other memorial service honoring the brave men and women who fought in U.S. wars.
☐Fly the United States flag.
☐Make a small donation to the Veterans of Foreign Wars and receive a red poppy in return.

❒Go to a local parade or watch one on television.
❒Walk through a flag-decorated cemetery.
❒Watch a televised ceremony at the tomb of the Unknown Soldier at Arlington National Cemetery.
❒Wear a red poppy on your lapel or collar.

In Flanders Fields
In Flanders fields the poppies blow
Between the crosses, row on row . . .
—John McCrae

Videos/DVDs

Be cautious when selecting modern videos for AD patients. Many are upset by currently accepted language, graphic sexuality and violence, preferring older films produced during their youth. Always read video/DVD content descriptions and check film ratings before renting or buying. Compare video and DVD prices at stores, online and through catalogs. Many are available at low- or discounted prices. Following are some films caregivers recommend.

❒Adventures:
    ❒*The African Queen* (Humphrey Bogart/ Katherine Hepburn) ❒*Barbary Coast* (Clark Gable) ❒*Ben Hur* (Charlton Heston) ❒Indiana Jones films ❒*Lost Horizon* (Ronald Coleman/Jane Wyatt) ❒*King Kong* (Fay Wray, 1933; Jeff

Bridges, 1976) ❑*Tarzan* series ❑*The Scarlet Pimpernel* (Leslie Howard) ❑*The Thief of Baghdad* (Douglas Fairbanks)

❑Animals:
❑Beethoven (the dog) movies ❑*Black Beauty* ❑*Fly Away Home* (Jeff Daniels/Anna Paquin) ❑*Homeward Bound* (Michael J. Fox/Sally Field) ❑*Lassie* series ❑*My Friend Flicka* (Roddy McDowell) ❑*National Velvet* (Elizabeth Taylor/ Mickey Rooney)

❑Animated cartoons:
❑Bugs Bunny ❑Casper the Friendly Ghost ❑Donald Duck ❑Little Lulu ❑Mr. Magoo ❑Mickey Mouse ❑Porky Pig ❑Sylvester ❑Tom and Jerry

❑Animated feature films, comedies and musicals:
❑*Bambi* ❑*Cinderella* ❑*Charley Brown* films ❑*101 Dalmations* ❑*The Lady and the Tramp* ❑*Roger Rabbit* ❑*Snow White and the Seven Dwarfs*

❑Comedies (early era):
❑Fatty Arbuckle ❑Clara Bow ❑W. C. Fields ❑Stan Laurel and Oliver Hardy ❑Little Rascals ❑Mae West. Old silent classics featuring ❑Ben Blue ❑Charlie Chaplin ❑Harold Lloyd ❑Buster Keaton ❑Marie Prevost ❑Hal Roach films ❑Ben Turpin

"Since he lost his hearing, Carl's favorite movies are the old silent film comedies, and I enjoy them, too."

☐Comedies (middle era) :
 ☐Bud Abbott and Lou Costello films ☐*Adams
 Rib* (Katherine Hepburn) ☐Bing Crosby/Bob
 Hope road pictures ☐*Father of the Bride*
 (Spencer Tracy) ☐*The Long, Long Trailer*
 (Lucille Ball/Desi Arnaz) ☐*The Egg and I* (Fred
 McMurray) ☐*Ma and Pa Kettle* series ☐Marx
 Brothers films ☐*Pat and Mike* (Katherine
 Hepburn/Spencer Tracy) ☐Three Stooges short
 features
☐Comedies (modern):
 ☐*Angels in the Outfield* ☐*The Bad News Bears*
 (Walter Matthau) ☐*City Slickers* (Billy Crystal)
 ☐*Father of the Bride* (Steve Martin/Diane
 Keaton) ☐*Hello, Dolly!* (Barbra Steisand)
 ☐*Home Alone* series (Macaulay Culkin) ☐*The
 Love Bug* (Dean Jones) ☐*Mr. Mom* (Michael
 Keaton/Teri Garr) ☐*Mrs. Doubtfire* (Robin
 Williams) ☐*The Santa Claus* (Tim Allen) ☐*Some
 Like It Hot* (Jack Lemon/Tony Curtis/Marilyn
 Monroe) ☐*Three Amigos* (Steve Martin/Chevy
 Chase) ☐*Three Men and a Baby* (Tom Selleck)
 ☐*Thoroughly Modern Milly* (Julie Andrews)
 ☐*Vacation* (Chevy Chase) ☐*Yours, Mine and
 Ours* (Lucille Ball/Henry Fonda)

❑Construction how-it's-done videos:
❑*Road Construction Ahead*, *House Construction Ahead*. Fred Levine Productions Co.
❑Drama:
❑*All That Heaven Allows* (Jane Wyman) ❑*The Best Years of Our Lives* (Myrna Loy) ❑*Boys Town* (Spencer Tracy) ❑*Dark Victory* (Bette Davis) ❑*Forever and a Day* (Merle Oberon) ❑*The Good Earth* (Paul Muni/Luise Reiner) ❑*Gone With the Wind* (Clark Gable/Vivien Leigh) ❑*Good Morning, Miss Dove* (Jennifer Jones) ❑*Mrs. Miniver* (Greer Garson) ❑*Pollyanna* (Jane Wyman) ❑*The Yearling* (Gregory Peck/Jane Wyman)
❑History (American) (NOTE: Older movies are generally less stressful because battle scenes are less graphic than those in modern films):
❑*Brigham Young—Frontiersman* (Tyrone Power/Linda Darnell) ❑*Friendly Persuasion* (Gary Cooper/Dorothy McGuire) ❑*The Grapes of Wrath* (Henry Fonda) ❑*Hawaii* (Richard Harris) ❑*How the West Was Won* (John Wayne) ❑*Little House on the Prairie* series ❑*North and South* (Patrick Swayze) ❑*Plymouth Adventure* (Gene Tierney/Spencer Tracy) ❑*Sergeant York* (Gary Cooper) ❑*Shenandoah* (James Stewart/Doug McClure) ❑*Texas* (William Holden/Glenn Ford) ❑*How the West Was Won* (John Wayne) ❑*The Westerner* (Gary Cooper)
❑Musicals:
❑*Annie Get Your Gun* (Betty Hutton/Howard

Keel) □*Auntie Mame* (Rosalind Russell) □*The Bells Are Ringing* (Judy Holiday/Dean Martin) □*Broadway Melody of 1936* (Eleanor Powell/Jack Benny) □*Fiddler on the Roof* (Topol) □*Glorifying the American Girl* (F. Ziegfeld, 1929) □*42nd Street* (Ruby Keeler) □*Gypsy* (Natalie Wood/Ethel Merman) □*The King and I* (Yul Brenner/Deborah Kerr) □*Mame* (Lucille Ball) □*My Fair Lady* (Rex Harrison) □*Oklahoma* (Gordon McCrae/Shirley Jones) □*Singing in the Rain* (Gene Kelly/Debbie Reynolds) □*The Sound of Music* (Julie Andrews) □*State Fair* (Jeannie Crane, 1945; Alice Faye/ Ann-Margaret, 1962) □*The Unsinkable Molly Brown* (Debbie Reynolds) □*Guys and Dolls* (Frank Sinatra) □*Seven Brides for Seven Brothers* (Jane Powell/Howard Keel) □*South Pacific* (Mitzi Gaynor) □*The Wizard of Oz* (Judy Garland)

> *"I like the old movies best, because I can watch them with my grandchildren and not feel embarrassed."*
> —Grandma Bea

□Religious:
□*A Man Called Peter* (Richard Todd) □*The Bells of St. Mary's* (Bing Crosby) □*Boys Town* (Spencer Tracy) □*David and Bathsheba* (Gregory Peck) □*The Egyptian* (Victor Mature), □*Esther and the King* (Joan Collins) □*King of Kings* (Jeffrey Hunter) □*Lights: The Miracle of Chanukah* (Judd Hirsch) □*Lilies of the Field*

(Sidney Poitier) ❏*Moses* (Ben Kingsley)
❏Shirley Temple movies. Originally in black and white, many are now available in colorized versions.
❏Sports:
> ❏*A League of Their Own* (Tom Hanks/Geena Davis) ❏*The Babe Ruth Story* (William Bendix) ❏*Eight Men Out* (John Cusack) ❏*The Jackie Robinson Story* (Jackie Robinson/Rubee Dee) ❏*Knute Rockney: All American* (Ronald Reagan/ Pat O'Brien) ❏*Jim Thorpe—All American* (Burt Lancaster)

❏TV Classics:
> ❏*The Flintstones* ❏*Green Acres* ❏*The Honeymooners* ❏*I Love Lucy* ❏*Lassie* ❏*The Lawrence Welk Show* ❏*Mayberry RFD* ❏ *Mr. Ed* ❏*Perry Mason* ❏*Petticoat Junction* ❏*Sgt. Bilko*, ❏*The Ed Sullivan Show* ❏*Your Show of Shows*

❏Westerns:
> Films featuring ❏Gene Autry ❏Bronco Billy ❏Hopalong Cassidy ❏The Cisco Kid ❏Roy Rogers and Dale Evans ❏Tom Mix ❏John Wayne ❏Zorro. ❏*Giant* (Elizabeth Taylor/Rock Hudson) ❏*Red River* (John Wayne) ❏*Son of Paleface* (Bob Hope comedy) ❏*The Way the West Was Won* (John Wayne/James Stewart) ❏*The Way West* (Kirk Douglas/Robert Mitchum)

"The greatest gift is a portion of thyself."
—Ralph Waldo Emerson

U.S. Movie History Highlights

1889 — First moving picture film is created by Thomas Edison on a base developed by John Eastman.

1891 — Thomas Edison files for first U.S. motion picture camera patent.

1896 — First films (brief scenes of dancing, ocean surf, and other activities) are shown on a public screen at Koster and Bial's Music Hall, New York City.

1903 — First film (silent) with a plot, *The Great American Train Robbery* (length 8 minutes) is released.

1905 — First nickelodeon theatre opens in Pittsburgh, Pennsylvania. Patrons pay a nickel to see a short film on a small screen.

1907 — The first public, color motion picture with sound is shown in Cleveland, Ohio. Footage includes scenes from an opera, a bullfight and a speech.

1909 — First notable animated film, *Gertie the Dinosaur*.

1912 — First screen subtitles explain action.

1922 — Technicolor process is perfected.

1927 — First talking movie, *The Jazz Singer* (Al Jolson).

1929 — First Oscar awards.

1938 — Disney releases *Snow White and the Seven Dwarfs*.

1939 — Blockbusters *The Wizard of Oz* (Judy Garland) and *Gone With the Wind* (Clark Gable and Vivian Leigh) open .

1954 — CinemaScope introduced in *The Robe*.

—Various sources

Visitors/Visiting

"Go often to the house of thy friend,
for weeds choke the unused path. "

—Ralph Waldo Emerson

☐Invite a friend or family member to call and visit you. **Caregiver**: Encourage adults, children and teenagers to call and visit frequently, and let them know that brief calls and visits are ideal.

❑ Go to a friend's or family member's home to visit. Take a photo album, collectible, or favorite project to share.

❑ Keep a list of people who call and visit. Put a check mark beside their names when they contact you and, perhaps, the date.

❑ Pose for snapshots with favorite people. **Caregiver**: Help your AD family member mount photos in an album and document names and dates.

❑ Send a thank-you card to someone who visits you.

George Washington's Birthday
(Born February 22, but now officially celebrated on the third Monday in February, Presidents' Day)

After America's thirteen colonies won independence, the birthday of the first president of the United States grew in popularity, replacing those days honoring Britain's king and queen. President Washington's birthday (February 22) was widely celebrated during his lifetime.

❑ Bake a cherry pie.

❑ Decorate the house with paper cutouts — red cherries, black tricorn hats, or pictures of George and Martha Washington. **Caregiver**:

Buy preprinted books of decorations or make your own.

❑Describe George Washington. What did he look like? Was he short or tall? What kind of clothes did he wear? What color was his hair? Were his teeth real or false?

❑Look through a pictorial history of George and Martha Washington and life in Virginia during the 1700s.

❑Put up, take down and fold the flag.

❑Read a story about George Washington.

❑Talk about the "I cannot tell a lie" story — which may or may not be true — when the youthful George Washington chopped down the family cherry tree.

❑Watch a video movie or television program about George Washington.

Weather Watch

"Red sky in the morning,
Sailors take warning,
Red sky at night,
Sailors delight."

❑Ask about and discuss family folklore and personal opinions about signs indicating weather changes. (e.g., an early or severe winter is indicated by larger amounts of nuts gathered by squirrels, or birds flying south early in the season; a storm is certain because the morning sky is pink; it will rain within three days because a frog is croaking.) **Caregiver**: Family folklore usually includes some great stories so be prepared to jot them down or tape record them for your family history files.

❑Monitor an indoor barometer.
❑Monitor a rain gauge.

> *"Uncle Ed often looks at a summer sky on a hot day and says he's worried we might get a 'blue norther.' Since we live in California where weather is stable, this seemed pretty silly. Then we learned that in Oklahoma where Ed grew up, storms called blue northers sometimes blow in on the heels of hot weather, and we realized Ed's comments were based on childhood memories."*

Weddings

Engagement parties, bridal showers, and weddings are exciting fare, especially for women. Encourage your family member to share in the joy of planning, organizing, and celebrating love.

❑Arrange a bouquet of flowers for an engagement party or bridal shower.
❑Assemble shower and wedding favors.

❑Attend an engagement party, bridal shower, or wedding.

❑Bake cookies for a bridal shower.

❑Browse through old photographs of family weddings. Discuss how the styles have changed from head to toe. What happy memories do you have of those weddings? Do you recall stories you were told about your parents' or grandparents' weddings? **Caregiver**: Document the names of people, relationships, dates, and interesting stories.

> *"This is a photograph of Mama and Daddy. They were married while sitting in the back of that horse-drawn buggy. That was very common in Oklahoma Territory around the turn of the century."*
> *—Vada*

> *"My great-grandfather wouldn't give his permission for his daughter Lila, my grandma, to marry the man she loved, so they eloped in 1910. They were married for over fifty years."*
> *—Marcella*

❑Buy a shower or wedding gift.

❑Buy a greeting card for an engagement, bridal shower or wedding.

❑Call and congratulate a newly engaged couple.

❑Decorate tables.

☐Describe your love life. How old were you when you were first kissed? Who did you kiss, or who kissed you? Did you have a lot of boyfriends or girlfriends? Where did you go on dates? Where did you meet your spouse? What did you like best about him or her? How old were you when you got engaged and married? Who is your sweetheart now?

☐Discuss weddings. What was your wedding like — small, large, simple, elegant? Where did your wedding take place — in a chapel, church, temple, home? What did you wear — long gown, afternoon dress, suit or tuxedo? Do you recall weddings you especially enjoyed — those of siblings, friends, relatives?

☐Fill candy bowls for celebrative events.

☐Pose for a picture with the bride and groom. **Caregiver**: Help your AD family member mount the snapshot in an album, recording names, date, and a brief note about the event.

☐Save napkins and other small souvenirs from engagement and wedding events and put them in your scrapbook or photo album.

☐Seal invitations.

☐Sort through a box of wedding memorabilia, and share stories about these old treasures.

☐Talk about honeymoons. Did you and your spouse go on a honeymoon? Where did you go? How did you get there? How long did you stay? Was it fun?

❏Tape a bow and greeting card on a gift.
❏Wrap a gift.

> **"Love comforteth like sunshine after rain."**
> **—William Shakespeare**

Wild, Wild West

How are yuh, there, cowboy?
I hope you are well.
Just light from your saddle
And rest fer a spell. . . .
—Curley W. Fletcher
Songs of the Sage, 1931

❏Collect western miniatures — cowboys, cattle, horses, lariets, saddles, Stetson hats, boots.
❏Create a collage using pictures cut from western magazines and catalogs.
❏Demonstrate your skill playing a guitar, banjo, harmonica, violin, saw, or other musical instrument.
❏Eat cowboy grub — bean soup with ham hock or bacon, beef stew, fried potatoes and onions, cornbread, biscuits, grits, fried pies, and other favorites.
❏Feed an apple, carrot, or sugar cube to a gentle horse.
❏Go to a rodeo.
❏Invite someone to play a banjo, fiddle, guitar or

harmonica for you.

☐Have lunch or dinner at a western-themed restaurant.

☐Listen to western music — Eddie Arnold, Sons of the Pioneers, Gene Autry, Roy Rogers, and other old classics.

☐Look at displays in a western-themed museum.

☐Subscribe to a magazine with a western theme — *American Cowboy*, *Cowboys & Country*, *Wild West*, or others.

☐Read a book or story about a western character or subject — Martha Jane "Calamity Jane" Canary Burke, Christopher "Kit" Carson, William "Buffalo Bill" Cody, Charles Jesse "Buffalo" Jones, Phoebe Anne "Annie" Oakley, James Butler "Wild Bill" Hickok; branding irons, cattle roping, buffalo, Longhorn cattle, mustangs, quarter horses, railroads, saddles, six-shooters, Texas Rangers, and others.

☐Relax at a horse show.

☐Ride on a horse or in a horse-drawn wagon.

☐Sing cowboy songs — *Buffalo Gals*, *Clementine*, *Down in the Valley*, *Home on the Range*, *Old Chisholm Trail*, and others.

☐Take a ride in a stagecoach.

☐Tour a frontier village.

☐Visit a horse or cattle ranch.

☐Watch a western movie. (*See video section for recommended films.*)

Women

Although they were significant, the accomplishments of women in American history were often overlooked in history books, and women's freedoms were extremely limited until recent years. You're sure to discover valuable insights into women's history by talking with your AD family member about past female experiences.

Women's Equality Day (August 26)

On August 26, 1920, the 19th Amendment to the U.S. Constitution granted women the right to vote. In 1971 the U.S. Congress designated August 26 as Women's Equality Day.

Women's History Month (March)

Through the efforts of the Women's History Project in California, and museums, libraries and educators across the country, the U.S. Congress in 1987 passed a resolution designating March as Women's History Month.

❑Attend a program focusing on important contributions to society by women.
❑(For women) Discuss your life as a female.

When you were growing up, how were girls expected to behave? What were you allowed to do that boys were not? What were boys allowed to do that you were not? What were you expected to do when you grew up — work outside the home, be a homemaker? What type work did women do in the home? What type careers did women have? Do you think women's lives were better in the old days or today?

☐Enjoy a fashion show featuring historic women's clothing.

☐Join with other women to reminisce about the past. Serve tea in pretty cups and elegant little cookies or cakes.

☐Mail a greeting card to a favorite woman.

☐Read a story or book about a famous woman — Clara Barton, Emily Dickinson, Althea Gibson, Georgia O'Keefe, Jacqueline Kennedy Onassis, Mary Pickford, Eleanor Roosevelt, Sojourner Truth, or others.

☐(For women) Record a story about your life experiences as a woman. **Caregiver**: Tape record, videotape or type your AD family member's stories for future generations. Contribute copies to The National Women's History Project archives.

☐Talk about women you have known. Who was your favorite? Why? Who was your least favorite?

☐Telephone a woman who is important to you
  and tell her you love and appreciate her.
☐Watch a movie about a significant woman or
  group of women.

Woodworking

*Woodworking projects are especially appealing to men.
I find it amazing that some AD men refuse to participate
in general craft activities, which they feel are too
feminine, but will eagerly tackle a woodworking project,
which they define as masculine. Women, on the other
hand, enjoy most activities without reservation.*

☐Apply decorative decals to wooden objects.
☐Build or help build easy projects: simple
  birdhouses, birdfeeders, planters, shelves, etc.
☐Collect and display small wooden boxes.
  Caregiver: Look for inexpensive boxes at
  discount stores, import shops, yard sales, thrift
  stores, and secondhand stores. Damaged boxes
  can be repaired, sanded, oiled, waxed, or
  varnished.
☐Collect and display small wooden objects —
  animal figures, cars, dolls, doll furniture,
  jewelry, rulers, spoons, toothpick holders,
  yo-yos, or others.
☐Decorate wood objects — birdhouses, small
  wall shelves, wall plaques, wreathes — with
  silk flowers, leaves, ivy, miniature fruit, veg-

etables and birds, silk butterflies, moss, or hand-painted designs.

❑Paint simple wood objects.

❑Sand wood, especially on already built projects.

❑Share a finished project with a child or teenager. **Caregiver**: If needed, assist your AD family member in explaining how the work was done.

❑Visit a craft store and select a wood project to work on, along with appropriate accessories.

"Chester spends many hours enthusiastically sanding birdhouses. While working, he talks about what color he plans to paint each house, where he'll hang it, and what birds will nest there, but he never does more than the sanding."

World War I (1914-1918)

People over 82 are most likely to remember events during this war, which was fought mainly in Europe and the Middle East. The United States entered the war in 1917. Currently, there are approximately 1,000 U.S. veterans of WWI still living.

❑Browse through memorabilia from WWI — family letters, newspaper clippings, military medals, war saving stamps, scrapbooks, photo albums. Why is each souvenir important to you?

❏Discuss home life during WWI. Did your family live in the country or in town? What did civilians do to aid the war effort – use corn instead of wheat? substitute fish and beans for meat? limit the amount of fats in cooking and soap-making? use syrups instead of sugar? Did your family eat less as the government requested and observe Meatless Mondays and Wheatless Wednesdays? Did you buy Victory Bonds, Liberty Bonds or War Savings Stamps? What factories in your area were converted to wartime uses? Do you recall the government introducing daylight saving time to save coal and oil?

❏Look through photos taken during WWI — military and home sites. Who are the people? What are they doing? What were their personalities?

❏Talk about WWI military experiences. Did you or any members of your family serve in the military during WWI? Did they fight in European or Middle Eastern battles?

> "War is not merely justifiable, but imperative, upon honorable men, upon an honorable nation, where peace can only be obtained by the sacrifice of conscientious conviction or of national welfare."
> —Theodore Roosevelt, 1906

```
┌─────────────────────────────────────────────────────┐
│              Key Participants in World War I          │
│                                                       │
│  Allies                        Central Powers         │
│  Belgium                       Austria-Hungary        │
│  France                        Bulgaria               │
│  Great Britain and countries of   Germany             │
│     the British Empire         Turkey                 │
│  Greece                                               │
│  Italy                                                │
│  Japan                                                │
│  Montenegro                                           │
│  Portugal                                             │
│  Rumania                                              │
│  Russia                                               │
│  Serbia                                               │
│  United States                                        │
└─────────────────────────────────────────────────────┘
```

World War II (1939-1945)

People over 55 are most likely to remember events during this war, which began in Europe in 1939, enjoined by the United States in 1941 when Japan bombed Pearl Harbor, and ended in 1945 with the surrender of Germany in May and Japan in September. There are more than 5 million WWII vets living in the U.S.

❑Browse through WWII memorabilia — letters, newspaper clippings, military medals, ration tickets, souvenir plates, dolls, decorative sofa pillows, lapel pins, service flags. Discuss a few of these unique items, one by one. When did you get this? Who did this belong to? What do you remember best about that time?

❑Discuss home life during WWII. Did you plant a victory garden? What did your family do during blackouts? What products were rationed? What products did you have the most difficulty buying — gasoline, tires, coffee, meat, sugar, cheese, canned food, butter, shoes, clothing, etc? How did you manage without these products? What did your family do on the home front to help the war effort — collect newspapers, metal, fat, rags; write letters and send baked goods to men and women in the armed forces; knit socks and mittens; buy savings bonds?

☐Discuss women's roles during WWII. Were you a homemaker, mother or sister of a military man or service woman — Army (WAC), Navy (WAVE), or Air Force (WAF) — or a defense plant employee ("Rosie the Riveter")?

☐Listen to WWII music. **Caregiver**: Big bands were popular, jive (a danceable form of jazz) was introduced. Dancers got their kicks from the jitterbug and the Lindy hop, which was a variation of the jitterbug.

☐Look through photos taken during WWII. Who are the people? What are they doing? Do you think those were good times or bad?

☐Read selections and look at the photos in journalist Tom Brokaw's books, *The Greatest Generation* and *The Greatest Generation Speaks*. **Caregiver**: These excellent books focus on the heroism and survival of the men and women who fought in World War II.

Yard Work

Stress-free work in the great outdoors is relaxing, gives men and women a sense of purpose and helps maintain muscle strength and flexibility.

☐ Carry debris to the garbage can.
☐ Edge the lawn.
☐ Hose the patio, deck, porch or walkway.
☐ Listen to upbeat music from a portable radio or tape player while you work.
☐ Mow the lawn.
☐ Paint a fence or outbuilding.
☐ Push a wheelbarrow.
☐ Put away tools, work gloves, and supplies.
☐ Rake leaves.
☐ Serve refreshments at break time.
☐ Shovel mud and debris from ditches.
☐ Stack firewood.
☐ Sweep spiderwebs from porch corners.
☐ Sweep walkways.

Yard Sales

Not everyone enjoys yard sales, but if you and your AD family member do, share the joy of bargain hunting or hosting your own event.

☐ Handcraft items to sell at a yard sale. **Caregiver**: (*See craft section for ideas.*) Encourage and help your family member to supervise sales at the table, answer questions, and enjoy compliments from shoppers.

☐Hand customers' cash for purchase to cashier and hand change back to customers.

☐Help plan, mark prices, or organize items for a yard sale.

☐Serve as the "yard-sale greeter." **Caregiver**: Give your AD family member a decorative "Greeter" or "Hi, I'm Ardith" name tag. Set a comfortable chair in a shady spot where yard sale visitors will pass by and let her pass out wrapped candies, cookies or small glasses of lemonade.

☐Spend an hour or two visiting nearby yard sales. **Caregiver**: Make sure your loved one has a few dollars to spend as he pleases. Take an interest in and don't criticize his purchases, whatever they may be. If it's something totally inappropriate, gently redirect him to other items.

> *"When Uncle Jim wanted to buy a dilapidated lawn mower at a yard sale, I agreed it was a very interesting find but pointed out that we live in a condominium and have no lawn. Then I suggested he choose one or two of the decorative pots, which would be perfect for our small patio. On the way home, we bought plants for Uncle Jim to plant in his pots."*

"At our neighbor's yard sale Mother bought several pieces of moth-eaten fabric 'to make a quilt for winter.' Although she no longer has the skills to sew, she spends many enjoyable hours folding and stroking the fabric and planning her quilt."

❑ Supervise an area containing familiar objects and answer questions about them during the sale.

❑ Tape prices on items to be sold.

Yom Kippur (Date varies)

The ten days beginning with Rosh Hashanah and ending with Yom Kippur are known as the Days of Awe.

Yom Kippur translates to the Day of Atonement and is probably the most important holy day of the Jewish year. Ten days after Rosh Hashanah, it is observed by fasting and a solemn religious service in which prayers seek forgiveness for sins and guidance to live righteously during the coming year. This is the last chance for forgiveness, for at the end of Yom Kippur, Almighty God closes the Book of Life until the following year. Yom Kippur usually occurs in September or October.

NOTE: <u>Do not</u> wish people a Happy Yom Kippur. It is not a happy holiday. It is, however, appropriate to say, "Have an easy fast."

The Day Before Yom Kippur
☐ Arrange candles.
☐ Bless your children.
☐ Enjoy honey cake.
☐ Feast on a sumptuous midday meal.
☐ Gather for the final, light meal in the evening.
   Caregiver: The traditional large, sumptuous midday meal and light evening meal prepare the worshiper for the fast that begins at sundown.
☐ Help prepare food for special meals.
☐ Light candles.
☐ Recite traditional special prayers.
☐ Wear plastic or canvas shoes or slippers, not leather.

On Yom Kippur
☐ Attend religious services.
☐ Avoid bathing, wearing leather shoes, marital relations and colognes, perfumes, lotions, etc.
☐ Avoid wearing gold jewelry.
☐ Fast. The fast is broken after evening services.
   Caregiver: Your family member should abstain from eating and drinking only if it is medically safe to do so.
☐ Light a *yahrzeit* ("year's time") *lamp*, a votive candle that will burn for over 24 hours.
   Caregiver: Special yahrzeit candles can be found in the kosher food section of grocery stores and in synagogue gift shops, but any

votive candle that will burn for over 25 hours will suffice.

☐Meditate on readings from the *Torah*.

☐Recite traditional special prayers.

☐Wear white clothes (optional). **Caregiver**: On Yom Kippur, Jews are compared to angels, but not all Jews opt to wear white.

> "Praise be to the Lord God, the God of Israel, who alone does marvelous deeds. Praise be to his glorious name forever; may the whole earth be filled with His glory."   —Psalm 73:18-19

❊ ❊ ❊

Epilogue

Shortly before this book was published, my father's physical and mental condition declined to the point where he needed 24-hour care by a healthcare team. After discussions with medical professionals, social workers, and other caregivers, and much soul-searching, many tears and abundant prayer, we released Dad into the gentle hands of professionals in a small, assisted-care home.

About the Author

B. J. FitzRay is a businesswoman, writer, editor, and consultant. A graduate of the University of California at Berkeley, she has enjoyed a successful and diverse career as a hospital patient representative and risk manager, newspaper columnist, and as a business entrepreneur. The mother of four adult children, B. J. lives with her husband, Norm, in northern California.

Selected Bibliography

Alzheimer's Disease at Time of Diagnosis. New York: Time/ Life Medical, Patient Education Media, Inc., 1996. Video.

Avadian, Brenda. *Where's My Shoes?* Lancaster, CA: North Star Books, 1999. (To order, call 1-800-852-4890.)

Brackey, Jolene. *Creating Moments of Joy for the Person with Alzheimer's or Dementia: A Journal for Caregivers.* West Lafayette: Purdue University Press, 2000.

Cordrey, Cindy. *Hidden Treasures: Music & Memory Activities for People with Alzheimer's.* Washington, D.C.: Center for Books on Aging. Serif Press, Inc., 1994. (To order, contact the publisher at 1-800-221-4272.)

Coughlan, Patricia Brown. *Facing Alzheimer's: Family Caregivers Speak.* New York: Ballantine, 1993.

Cowley, Geoffrey. "Alzheimer's: Unlocking the Mystery." *Newsweek* (January 31, 2000) 46-51.

Doernberg, M. *Stolen Mind: The Slow Disappearance of Ray Doernberg.* Chapel Hill, N.C.: Algonquin, 1989.

Goodwin, Dennis. *The Activity Director's Treasure Chest.* Kissimmee: The Activity Factory. (To order, contact the publisher at 1551 Key Court, Kissimmee, FL 32743.)

Honel, R. W. *Journey with Grandpa: Our Family's Struggle with Alzheimer's Disease.* Johns Hopkins University Press, 1988.

Kalb, Claudia. "Coping with the Darkness." *Newsweek* (January 31, 2000) 52-54.

Lemonick, Michael D. and Alice Park Mankato. "Alzheimer's: The Nun Study." *Time Magazine* (May 14, 2001) 54-64.

Mace, Nancy L. and Peter V. Rabins. *The 36-Hour Day.* Baltimore: The John Hopkins University Press, 1991.

Marcell, Jacqueline. *Elder Rage —or— Take My Father ... Please!: How to Survivie Caring for Aging Parents.* Irvine, CA: Impressive Press, 2001.

Meyer, Maria M. and Paula Derr. *The Comfort of Home*. Portland: CareTrust Publications LLC, 1998.

Nelson, James Lindemann and Hilde Lindermann Nelson. *Alzheimer's: Answers to Hard Questions for Families*. New York: Doubleday, 1996.

Rothert, Gene. *The Enabling Garden: Creating Barrier-Free Gardens*. Dallas: Taylor Publishing Co., 1994.

Shanks, Lela Knox. *Your Name Is Hughes Hannibal Shanks, A Caregiver's Guide to Alzheimer's*. Lincoln: University of Nebraska Press, 1996.

Sheridan, Carmel. *Failure-Free Activities for the Alzheimer's Patient*. San Francisco: Cottage Books, 1987. (To order, contact the publisher at 1-800-909-2673.

Snowdon, David. *Aging with Grace: What the Nun Study Teaches Us About Leading Longer, Healthier and More Meaningful Lives*. New York: Bantam, 2001.

Warner, Mark L. *The Complete Guide to Alzheimer's Proofing Your Home*. West Lafayette: Purdue University Press, 2000.

Yeomans, Kathleen. *The Able Gardener: Overcoming Barriers of Age & Physical Limitations*. Pownal: Storey Communications, Inc., 1992.

Zgola, Jitka M. *Doing Things*. Baltimore: The John Hopkins University Press, 1987.

Resources for Alzheimer's Disease Information

•**Alzheimer's Association**
919 N. Michigan Avenue
Suite 1100
Chicago, IL 60611-1676
(800) 272-3900; (312) 335-8700
fax (312) 335-1110
www.alz.org

•**Alzheimer's Disease Education and Referral Center**
P.O. Box 8250
Silver Spring, MD 20907
(800) 438-4380
adear@alzheimers.org

•**Traditional and alternative treatments of memory loss**
www.seniormemoryloss.com

•**Alzheimer's Disease International**
www.alz.co.uk

Stages of Alzheimer's Disease

The Functional Stages of Alzheimer's Disease and Their Incorporation into the Functional Assessment Staging (FAST) scale[1]

Stage	Clinical Diagnosis	Characteristics
1	Normal adult	No decline in function
2	Normal older adult	Personal awareness of functional decline
3	Early AD	Deficits noticed in demanding employment situations
4	Mild AD	Requires assistance in complicated tasks, such as handling finances, planning dinner party
5	Moderate AD	Requires assistance in choosing proper attire
6	Moderately severe AD	
6a		Requires assistance dressing
6b		Requires assistance bathing properly
6c		Requires assistance with mechanics of toileting
6d		Urinary incontinence
6e		Fecal incontinence
7	Severe AD	
7a		Speech ability limited to about a half-dozen intelligible words
7b		Intelligible vocabulary limited to a single word
7c		Ambulatory ability lost
7d		Ability to sit up lost
7e		Ability to smile lost
7f		Ability to hold up head lost

[1]Adapted from Reisberg, B. Functional assessment staging (FAST). Psychopharmacology Bulletin. 1988; 24 653-659. © 1984 by Barry Reisberg, M.D. All rights reserved.

Product Resources

Contact the following companies and Websites for catalogs and product information. Please note that requesting catalogs from any company may result in your name being added to their mailing list, or your name and address sold or given to other companies. If you do not want to receive unsolicited literature, specifically request that your name be limited to this one-time use only.

Please note that product prices may vary and include sales tax depending on where the item is purchased. In addition, if ordering by mail, shipping and handling charges will probably be added. We recommend calling vendors for prices and ordering information before sending checks.

We invite companies to send us information, catalogs, and samples of products considered appropriate for possible inclusion in future editions of this book. Forward information to the publisher at the following address.

Rayve Productions
P.O. Box 726
Windsor, CA 95492
rayvepro@aol.com
1-707-838-6200

Product Resource Suppliers

Contact the following for catalogs and product information.

•**The American Safety Razor Co.**
P.O Box 500
Staunton, VA 24402-0500
1-540-248-8000

•**Audubon Workshop**
The Wild Bird Specialists
5200 Schenley Place
Lawrenceburg, IN 47025
To order: 1-812-537-3583
Questions: 1-812-537-8628
fax 1-812-537-5108
www.AudubonWorkshop.com

•**Boyds Mills Press**
815 Church Street
Honesdale, PA 18431

•**Crossings Press**
Book Club Service Center
6550 E. 30th Street
P.O. Box 6325
Indianapolis, IN 46206-6325
317-541-8920
www.Crossings.com

•**Current, Inc.**
Express Processing Center
Colorado Springs, CO 80941-0001
1-800-848-2848
fax 1-800-993-3232
www.currentcatalog.com

•**Discovery Toys Inc.**
P.O. Box 5023
Livermore, CA 94551-5023
1-800-426-4777
www.discoverytoysinc.com

•**Elder Press**
The Alzheimer's Bookshelf
P.O. Box 490
Forest Knolls, CA 94933
1-800-909-2673 (COPE)
www.ElderBooks.com
info@ElderBooks.com

•**Fred Levine Productions Co.**
64 Main Street
Montpelier, VT 05602
1-800-843-3686
fax 1-802-229-6920
www.littlehardhats.com

•**Greg Markim Inc.**
Box 13245
Milwaukee, WI 53213
1-800-453-1485
www.arnoldgrummer.com

•**Henry Ford Museum**
1-313-982-6100 X2323
fax 1-313-982-6241
RETAIL@HFMGV.ORG

•**Inspirations (A division of Oriental Trading Co, Inc.)**
P.O. Box 2654
Omaha, NE 68103-2654
1-800-228-2269
www.oriental.com

•**National Women's History Project**
3343 Industrial Drive, Suite 4
Santa Rosa, CA 95403
707-636-2888
www.nwhp.org

•**Oriental Trading Co, Inc.**
P.O. Box 2654
Omaha, NE 68103-2654
1-800-228-2269
www.oriental.com

•**Rayve Productions Inc.**
P.O. Box 726
Windsor, CA 95492-9466
1-800-852-4890
www.rayveproductions.com
rayvepro@aol.com

•**Smithsonian National Air and Space Museum Bookstore**
Information Management Div.
7th St. & Independence Ave. SW
Washington, DC 20560
1-202-287-3480
www.smithsonianstore.com

•**Sourcebooks**
P.O. Box 4410
Naperville, IL 60567-4410
1-630-961-3900
fax 1-630-961-2168

•**Super Duper Productions**
Dept. SD 2000
P.O. Box 24997
Greenville, SC 29616-2497
1-800-277-8737
fax 1-800-978-7379
www.superduperinc.com
custserv@superduperinc.com

•**United Nations Publications Bookshop**
First Avenue & 46th Street
New York, New York 10017
1-800-553-3210
fax 1-212-963-4910
www.un.org/Pubs/bookshop
bookshop@un.org

•**Warren's Educational Supplies**
980 W. San Bernadino Rd.
Covina, CA 91722

•**YesterMusic (A Division of The Good Music Co.)**
Dept. 404590
P.O. Box 645
Holmes, PA 19043-0645
1-800-292-3800
www.yestermusic.com

Product Resources

Key: **A**...audiotape/CD; **B**...book; **b**...booklet; **C**...catalog; **G**...game; **M**...music; **V**...videotape; **W**...Website; **O**...other

Activity Books

You will find many children's activity books that appeal to women. Finding appropriate books for men is more challenging.

b •**Sticker books** ideal for men: *Tractors* (Item #SB001) and *Trucks* (Item SB002), $6.95 each. Little Hardhats. **Fred Levine Productions Co.**

b •**Dot-to-dots, mazes & hidden pictures** ideal for men: *All Around the Fire Station* (Item #AB002); *On the Construction Site* (Item #AB001); *What's in the Big Red Barn?* (#AB004). $4.95 each. Little Hardhats. **Fred Levine Productions Co.**

Airplanes/Aviation

B The following books and videos may be found through Websites such as Amazon.com and in bookstores or from the publisher where indicated.

V •*Biography: Amelia Earhart* by Nancy Shore. NY: Chelsea House Publishers. $12.99.

V •*Dreams of Flight, Smithsonian Air and Space Museum.* Early days of manned flight series. Videos, $11.50-12.99.

V •*Afterburner Boogie.* Jets in action, 45 min., video, $11.98.

V •*American Experience series* — **Lindbergh**. Video, $21.49.

V •*Cleared for Takeoff* — Airplanes and a cross-country flight. Produced for children but also appealing to adults, especially men. Lots of action. (Item #VID003) 30-47 minutes, $14.95 each. **Fred Levine Productions Company**

V   •*Flyers: In Search of a Dream*. Chronicles of the black flying experience. Video, $16.99.

V   •*Lindbergh's Great Race*. Video, $16.99

V   •*National Museum of Naval Aviation Tour*. Video, $16.99

V   • *The Ultimate Air Show*. Historic wingwalkers, the Thunderbirds, British Red Arrows, and Canadian Snowbirds. Video, $16.99

V   •*United States Air Force Museum*. Charlton Heston narrates this look at Air Force history in the Air Force museum. Video, $16.99.

Alzheimer's Survival Kits

O/   •Kits, baskets or boxes filled based on a subject or theme.
W   Designed to provide Alzheimer's patients with structured or diversional activities. $60-75. **Pro-Active Eldercare.** **www.proactiveeldercare.com/boxes.htm**

American History

B   •*The Greatest Generation,* $24.95, and *The Greatest Generation Generation Speaks: Letter and Reflections,* $19.95, by Tom Brokaw. Stories about Americans whose WWII sacrifices changed the course of history.

V   •*Little House on the Prairie*. Life on America's Great Plains. This set of five videotapes of the popular TV series includes the premiere movie and the marriage of Laura Ingalls. About $50/set of 5.

B   •*Our Century of Change* by the editors of *LIFE Magazine*. Superb photos reveal American life from 1900 to 2000. Elders will remember hearing about or living through the various eras; younger folks will enjoy discoveries about the "old days." $60 or less through discount resources.

B   •*Our Century in Pictures* compiled by the editors of *LIFE Magazine*. More than 750 photographs from *LIFE Magazine's* archives and insightful essays focus on the past century. $60 or less through discount resources.

B/
A
•*We Interrupt This Broadcast, 2nd edition, The Events That Stopped Our Lives...from the Hindenburg Explosion to the Death of John F. Kennedy Jr.* Includes two audio CDs and a comprehensive 10¾ x 10¼, 170-page book with numerous photographs. $49.95. **Sourcebooks**

Automobiles/Transportation

V
•*Auto Biography: Henry Ford and the Automobile in American Life.* Rare footage, historic photos and film. Video, $19.95. **Henry Ford Museum**

V
•*Video Tour of the Henry Ford Museum and Greenfield Village.* Interviews, historic film footage. Visit homes and workplaces of Thomas Edison, the Wright brothers, Noah Webster, and Henry Ford. Many original inventions and artifacts. Video, 30 min., $19.95. **Henry Ford Museum**

B
•*Link Across America, The Story of the Historic Lincoln Highway* by Mary E. Anderson. Children's book about America's first coast-to-coast highway. Contains numerous illustrations and photographs, map of original Lincoln Highway, cities along the route. $15.95. **Rayve Productions Inc.**

B
•*Verse by the Side of the Road,* under $10. A compilation of the humorous rhymes on Burma Shave signs along America's roadways. **The American Safety Razor Company**

Birds and Butterflies

The following products are available at libraries, bookstores, online and directly through publishers or distributors where indicated. For reduced rates, check out Crossings Press and Websites such as Amazon.com.

B
•*Amazing Butterflies* by John Still, photos by Jerry Young. (ages 4-8) Beautiful photographs and amazing facts. 1991, under $10.

B
•*Attracting Birds and Butterflies* by Barbara Ellis. (Ages 4-8)1997, under $15.

B   •*Bird and Butterfly Gardens* by Warren Schultz. 1997, under $12.

V   •*Bluebirds Up Close* video, 50 minutes, $29.95.
The Audubon Workshop.

O   •**Butterfly and Hummingbird Flower Seed Mix**, $6.99.
The Audubon Workshop.

O   •**Butterfly feeder and nectar.** The Audubon Workshop.

b   •*Enjoying Bluebirds More*, 32-page booklet, $4.95.
The Audubon Workshop.

b   •*Enjoying Butterflies More*, 32-page booklet, $4.95.
The Audubon Workshop.

B   •*Stoke's Bird Gardening Book* by Donald Stokes. $13.
Crossings Press.

B   •*Stoke's Butterfly Book* by Donald Stokes, $12.95.
Crossings Press.

B   • *Where Butterflies Grow* by Joanne Ryder (ages 4-8) 1996, under $7.

C/   •**Bird houses, nesting boxes, kits, bird foods, bird baths,**
O   **books, videos.** Colorful **catalog** contains many bird
photos and useful information. **The Audubon Workshop.**

Candy Recipes

B   •*Nancy's Candy Cookbook, How to Make Candy at Home
the Easy Way* by Nancy Shipman. $14.95. The author is a
professional candy maker and teacher. This book contains
dozens of excellent and easy recipes, including some that
require no cooking. **Rayve Productions Inc.**

Cards, Crafts, Games, Kits

The following companies carry many fun products and projects.
Log onto their Websites to review and evaluate items, or contact
them for catalogs.

C   •**Elder Press**

C   •**Oriental Trading Co, Inc.**

C   •**Super Duper Productions**
Super Duper's catalog is targeted to speech-language
pathologists and teachers, but you'll find many excellent
products appropriate for your AD family member or patient.
**Best sections for AD patients: "Language Cards" and
"Language Games" **Warren's Educational Supplies**

Chinese New Year

B   •*Celebrating the Lunar New Year: Great Things to Do in
the Classroom and at Home*, $6.95. This book contains
reproducible coloring sheets and templates for zodiac
animals, lion, dragon parade, Chinese words, and more.

O/
W   •*Lucky Plants*   **www.luckyplants.com**

W   •**Internet Lunar New Year Resources** (Legends, arts and
crafts, gifts, and foods)
www.familyculture.com/newyear_resources.htm

Christmas Pins & other holiday crafts

C   •**Inspirations catalog, Oriental Trading Company**
C   •**Sensational Crafts catalog, Oriental Trading Company**

House & Road Construction, Fire & Rescue

V   •**Road Construction Ahead** (Item #VID001)
V   •**House Construction Ahead** (Item #VID004)
V   •**Fire & Rescue** (Item #VID002)
V   •**Where the Garbage Goes** (Item #VID005)

Fine film production, accurate information, many
machines, lots of action. Ideal for men. 30-47 minutes.
$14.95 each. **Fred Levine Productions Company**

Dolls

B   •*Patty Reed's Doll: The Story of the Donner Party* by
Rachel K.Laurgaard. A wooden doll (a real doll now in a
museum) recalls the hope with which a group of pioneers
begins their journey and the ordeals they face as they travel
from Springfield, Illinois, to California. Wonderful
historical fiction for all ages. 143 pp., under $10.

B   *Stories of Little Girls and Their Dolls, Classics from an Age of Remembered Joy*, compiled by William C. Carroll. This book is a delightful compilation of illustrated doll stories from *St. Nicholas* magazine — 1873 to 1939, 8½ x 11, 175 pp., $19.95 or less. **Boyds Mills Press**

Farming

V   •**Farm Country Ahead** (Item #VID006)
V   **Fred Levine Productions Company**

Fishing Game

G   Available through WalMart and elsewhere. A **Pressman Corporation** product.

Fuzzy Postcards

O   •Available at many stores. Produced by **Super Duper Publications**

Greeting Cards, Name Stamps & more

C   •**Current, Inc.**

Japanese New Year

W   •Type **keywords "Japanese New Year"** or go to **www.jin.jcic.or.jp/today/culture/culture2.html**

Jewish Holidays & Judaism

W   •Glossary of Passover terms, traditional Seder recipes, and downloadable prayer books: **www.jewish.com/passover**

W   •View lyrics and listen to traditional music, and send virtual greeting cards: **www.holidays.net/passover**

Martin Luther King, Jr.

O   •Do Something Kindness & Justice Challenge

W   **Do Something**
Attn: Kindness & Justice Challenge
423 W. 55th St., 8th Floor
New York, NY 10019
www.coach.dosomething.org

This program is designed for school children but many of the suggested activities can be adapted for Alzheimer patients.

V/   •*Martin Luther King, Jr. Commemorative Collection*
W   *Video: A Life History of Dr. Martin Luther King*, **Jr.**
Available through bookstores and the Martin Luther King, Jr. Website bookstore. $30.
www.thekingcenter.org

Memory Boxes

O   •Shadow boxes can be found at craft stores and pictures frame shops. For convenience and durability, choose shadow boxes with deeper shelves and glass- or plastic-covered fronts that will protect contents from dust and ultraviolet (UV) rays.

Military

W   •**Veterans of Foreign Wars**
www.vfw.org

O   •**VFW Magazine**
Sharon Bowden
406 W. 34tth Street
Kansas City, MO 64111
1-816-756-3390
fax 1-816-968-1169
(Non-member subscriptions: $10/year U.S.; $15 other countries)

O   •**Operation Dear Abby:** December holiday season cards and letters to men and women of the Armed Forces, 13 oz. or less, Mid-November—January.

Any Service Member
Operation Dear Abby
Europe and South West Asia
APO AE 09135

Any Service Member
Operation Dear Abby
Mediterranean Basin
FPO AE 09646

Any Service Member
Operation Dear Abby
Far East
APO AE 96285

Any Service Member
Operation Dear Abby
Pacific Basin
FPO AE 95385

Music

**M/
A**
•*Best Loved Songs of the American People*. Contains 200 popular songs — from Irving Berlin tunes, to the *Star Spangled Banner*, to *The Impossible Dream*. $12.95. **Crossings Press**

**M/
A**
•*The Best of Glenn Miller*. 24 popular hits — *In the Mood, A String of Pearls, Don't Sit Under the Apple Tree, That Old Black Magic, Tuxedo Junction*, and more. 2 cassettes $12.98; CD $16.98. **YesterMusic**

**M/
A**
•*Big Band Music*. Includes 37 superstars — Count Basie, Benny Goodman, Woody Herman, Artie Shaw, Tommy Dorsey and other musicians of the big band era. 4 one-hour cassettes, $21.95. **Elder Press**

**M/
A**
•*Malt Shop Memories*. 36 hits of the 1950's by the original artists — *Dream Lover, Earth Angel, Sh Boom, April Love, Sea of Love, Venus, Mr. Sandman, My Special Angel*, and more. 2 cassettes $19.98; 2 CDs $26.98. **YesterMusic**

**O/
A**
•*Old Time Radio*. Radio drama, newscasts, comedy, and popular radio commercials. Packed with entertainment, adventure and nostalgia. 4 one-hour cassettes, $21.95. **Elder Press**

**M/
A**
•*Sentimental Journey*. 44 big band hits by the original artists — *In the Mood, Dancing in the Dark, One O'clock Jump, Star Dust, Blues in the Night*, and more. 3 cassettes $19.95; 2 CDs $24.95. **YesterMusic**

M/ •*Sioux City Sue*. 42 World War II jukebox favorites with a
A   western flavor, by the original artists — *Bouquet of Roses,*
    Tennessee Waltz, Tumbling Tumbleweeds, Cold, Cold
    Heart, Cool Water, Pistol Packin' Mama, Candy Kisses,
    and more. 3 cassettes $19.95; 2 CDs $24.95.
    YesterMusic

M/ •*White Cliffs of Dover*. 42 World War II love songs by the
A   original artists — *Always, Seems Like Old Times, I'll Be*
    Seeing You, Harbor Lights, Serenade in Blue, Deep
    Purple, and more. 3 cassettes $19.95; 2 CDs $24.95.
    YesterMusic

M/ •*The Wonderful 30's*. 50 memorable songs by the original
A   artists — *Did You Ever See a Dream Walking?, All I Do*
    Is Dream of You, On the Sunny Side of the Street, Two
    Sleepy People, Easter Parade, Jeepers Creepers, Smoke
    Gets in Your Eyes, Stormy Weather, My Baby Just Cares
    for Me, and more. 2 cassettes $34.95; 3 CDs $39.95.
    YesterMusic

Papermaking Kits & Books

O   •**Greg Markim Inc.**

Playful Patterns

G   •**Discovery Toys**

Puzzles

Simple puzzles are readily available at many stores. The
following easy-grip wood puzzles have masculine themes:

G   •**Construction Vehicles** (Item #CP005)
G   •**Farm** (Item #FP02)
G   •**Fire Truck** (Item #FT04)
G   •**Tools** (Item #CT006; Transportation (Item #TP03)
G   •**Vehicles** (Item #VP01). $10.95 each
    Fred Levine Productions Company

Science

W   •Online, type **keyword: World of Science**

Silent Movies

C   •**silentsaregolden.com**
       Listing of more than 750 silent movies on video plus
       photos, reviews and other information.

C   •**VIDEOBRARY** (catalogs available)
       5812 Wish Avenue
       Encino, CA 91316
       323-660-0187
       323-660-5571

Women

C   •**National Women's History Project**

World War II

B   •*Our Finest Hour* by the editors of *LIFE Magazine*.
       Excellent photographs detail the courage and heroism of
       World War II from beginning battles to happy homecom-
       ings. Color and black and white photos. $29.95 or less
       through discount resources.

Index

BOOKS & MUSIC FROM RAYVE PRODUCTIONS

CAREGIVING / PARENTING / COUNSELING

•*ALZHEIMER'S ACTIVITIES, Volume 1, Hundreds of Activities for Men and Women with Alzheimer's Disease and Related Disorders* by B.J. FitzRay, ISBN 1-877810-80-0, hardcover, $23.95

•*ALZHEIMER'S ACTIVITIES, Volume 2, More Activities for Men and Women with Alzheimer's Disease and Related Disorders* by B.J. FitzRay, ISBN 1-877810-81-9, hardcover, $24.95

•*WHEN A PARENT GOES TO JAIL, A Comprehensive Guide for Counseling Children of Incarcerated Parents* by Rebecca M. Yaffe and Lonnie F. Hoade, for counseling ages 5-14, ISBN 1-877810-08-8, $49.95; companion workbook, ISBN 1-877810-11-8, $29.95

•*JOY OF READING, A Family's Fun-filled Guide to Reading Success* by Debbie Duncan, ISBN 1-877810-45-2, $14.95

•*WHEN MOLLY WAS IN THE HOSPITAL, A Book for Brothers and Sisters of Hospitalized Children* by Debbie Duncan, ages 3-12, ISBN 1-877810-44-4, hardcover $12.95

HISTORY

•*20 TALES OF CALIFORNIA, A Rare Collection of Western Stories* by Hector Lee, ages 14-adult, ISBN 1-877810-62-2, softcover, $9.95

•*LINK ACROSS AMERICA, A Story of the Historic Lincoln Highway* by Mary Elizabeth Anderson, ages 6-13, ISBN 1-877810-97-5, hardcover, $15.95

•*BUFFALO JONES, The Man Who Saved America's Buffalo* by Carol A. Winn, illustrated by William J. Geer, ages 10-14, ISBN 1-877810-30-4, hardcover, $12.95

•*WINDSOR, THE BIRTH OF A CITY, A History and Case Study of the People, Dynamics and Processes* by Gabriel A. Fraire, ISBN 1-877810-91-6, hardcover, $21.95

CHILDREN'S / YOUNG ADULT

•*NEKANE, THE LAMINA & THE BEAR, A Tale of the Basque Pyrenees* by Frank P. Araujo, Ph.D., illustrated by Xiao Jun Li, ages 6-10, ISBN 1-877810-01-0, hardcover $30.00, Limited-quantity collectible.

•*THE PERFECT ORANGE, A Tale from Ethiopia* by Frank P. Araujo, Ph.D., illustrated by Xiao Jun Li, ages 4-13, ISBN 1-877810-94-0, hardcover, $16.95

•*NIGHT SOUNDS (bedtime story)* by Lois G. Grambling, illustrated by Randall F. Ray, ages 4-6, ISBN 1-877810-77-0, hardcover, $12.95; ISBN 1-877810-83-5, softcover, $6.95

•*LOS SONIDOS DE LA NOCHE (*Spanish edition of *NIGHT SOUNDS)* by Lois G. Grambling, illustrated by Randall F. Ray, ages 4-6, ISBN 1-877810-76-2, hardcover, $12.95; ISBN 1-877810-82-7, softcover, $6.95

•*THE LAUGHING RIVER, A Folktale for Peace* by Elizabeth Vega, illustrated by Ashley Smith, ages 5-12; book: ISBN 1-877810-35-5, hardcover, $16.95; musical audiotape: ISBN 1-877810-36-3, $9.95; book & musical audiotape combo: ISBN 1-877810-37-1, $23.95

•*WHEN MOLLY WAS IN THE HOSPITAL, A Book for Brothers and Sisters of Hospitalized Children* by Debbie Duncan, ages 3-12, ISBN 1-877810-44-4, hardcover $12.95

•*LINK ACROSS AMERICA, A Story of the Historic Lincoln Highway* by Mary Elizabeth Anderson, ages 6-13, ISBN 1-877810-97-5, hardcover, $15.95

•*BUFFALO JONES, The Man Who Saved America's Buffalo* by Carol A. Winn, illustrated by William J. Geer, ages 10-14, ISBN 1-877810-30-4, hardcover, $12.95

•*NICKY JONES AND THE ROARING RHINOS* by Lois G. Grambling, illustrated by William J. Geer, ages 6-8, ISBN 1-877810-14-2, softcover, $6.95

•*SHOW ME A SIGN, A Baby's Guide to Sign Language* by Cynthia R. Thomas, M.S., CCC-SLP, ages 2-6, ISBN 1-877810-78-9, hardcover, $14.95

PERSONAL HEIRLOOM-QUALITY JOURNAL

•*LIFETIMES, THE LIFE EXPERIENCES JOURNAL,* heirloom quality, over 150 categories, ISBN 1-877810-34-7, hardcover, gilt-edged pages, $49.95

COOKBOOK

•*NANCY'S CANDY COOKBOOK, Second Edition, How to Make Candy at Home the Easy Way* by Nancy Shipman, ISBN 1-877810-64-9, softcover, $15.95

BUSINESS & CAREER

•*THE INDEPENDENT MEDICAL TRANSCRIPTIONIST,*
*4th edition, The Comprehensive Guidebook for Career Success
in a Home-based Medical Transcription Business* by Donna
Avila-Weil, CMT & Mary Glaccum, CMT, ISBN 1-877810-52-5,
softcover, $39.95

•*INDEPENDENT MEDICAL CODING, The Comprehensive
Guidebook for Career Success as a Medical Coder* by Donna
Avila-Weil, CMT & Rhonda Regan, CCS, ISBN 1-877810-17-7,
softcover, $34.95

•*NATIONWIDE MEDICAL TRANSCRIPTION SERVICE
DIRECTORY 2000, The Most Comprehensive Published Listing of Medical Transcription Service Professionals in the U.S.*
compiled by Denise Schultheis, MT, ISBN 1-877810-88-6,
softcover, $39.95

•*SMART TAX WRITE-OFFS, 4th edition, Hundreds of Tax
Deduction Ideas for Home-based Businesses, Independent
Contractors, All Entrepreneurs* by Norm Ray, CPA, ISBN 1-
877810-21-5, softcover, $14.95

•*EASY FINANCIALS FOR YOUR HOME-BASED BUSINESS,
The Time-saving, Money-saving Small Business Handbook* by
Norm Ray, CPA, ISBN 1-877810-92-4, softcover, $19.95

•*SHRINKING THE GLOBE INTO YOUR COMPANY'S
HANDS, The Step-by-Step International Trade Guide for Small
Businesses* by Sidney R. Lawrence, PE, ISBN 1-877810-46-0,
softcover, $24.95

MEDICAL REFERENCE

•*INTERNAL MEDICINE WORDS, More than 8000 Words,
Terms, and Quick Definitions* compiled by medical
transcriptionist Minta Danna, ISBN 1-877810-68-1, softcover,
$29.95

ORDER

For mail orders, please complete this order form and forward with check, money order or credit card information to Rayve Productions, POB 726, Windsor CA 95492. If paying with a credit card, you can call us toll-free at 800.852.4890 or fax this completed form to Rayve Productions at 707.838.2220.

You can also order at our Website at www.rayvepro.com.

❐ Please send me the following book(s):

Title _____ Price ____ Qty. ____ Amount _____

Title _____ Price ____ Qty. ____ Amount _____

Title _____ Price ____ Qty. ____ Amount _____

Title _____ Price ____ Qty. ____ Amount _____

Quantity Discount: 4 items →10%; **7 items →15%; 10 items →20%**	Subtotal $ ____
	Discount $ ____
	Subtotal $ ____
Sales Tax: Californians please add 7.75% sales tax	Sales Tax $ ____
Shipping:	Shipping $ ____
Book rate — $4 for first book + $1 each additional Priority — $5 for first book + $1 each additional	Total $ ____

Name_____ Phone_____

Address _____

City State Zip _____

❐Check enclosed $ _____   Date _____

❐Charge my Visa/MC/Discover/AMEX $ _____

Credit card # _____Exp. _____

Signature_____ *Thank you!* _{Alz01}